What people are saying:

"Healing from the Heart is an important contribution to the humanization of health care. I would definitely link patient safety and quality to the importance of health care providers learning this process."

Dr. Nancy Moore, Sr. VP Healing Health Services,
Chief Nursing Officer, St. Charles Medical Center, Redmond, OR

....

"Tim Dawes's work, *Healing from the Heart…* is a rare jewel of a book packed with practical ideas and a powerful model for making empathy more transparent to patients and their families. Use this model and practical guidelines and watch your Patient Satisfaction scores climb."

Chris Ibanez, Manager, Training and Development,
Overlake Hospital Medical Center, Bellevue, WA

....

"Healing from the Heart, by Timothy Dawes, is the antidote for what's missing in nursing education. Here, he gives us a systematic approach that you can use to deal with any patient situation. Using an empathetic perspective, you will learn to view every patient's call for help from the vantage point of what you intend to give them. The result is less frustration for you, more satisfaction for them, and a new found joy in the work!"

RN (publishers of the Journal and RNWeb)

....

"Mr. Dawes has provided a valuable tool for caregivers to understand and improve communications. Our patients increasingly expect no less than excellence in communication and *Healing from the Heart* provides a process for health care providers to achieve this worthy goal."

American College of Physician Executives

"Healing from the Heart...is an excellent resource for both those starting in healthcare and those who have been immersed in the continuum for some time. I found the practical approach for the ALIVE Model works in all areas, not just direct patient care but also in case management, business and our own personal lives."

American Association of Managed Care Nurses

....

"Timothy Dawes' new book, *Healing from the Heart*, is unlike anything I have seen before… a step-by-step guide to relating empathetically with people around you. I enthusiastically recommend it as a tool for Direct Support staff and for managers. The book is easy to use, filled with practical exercises that cement his points, and eminently practical. Dawes helps to unpack the hidden messages and emotion from our everyday language and offers clear and applicable strategies to improve our communication and rapport."

Michael R. McCoy, Ph.D., Executive Director, California Rehabilitation Association

....

"This is a well laid out, simply written, and very practical tool to aid clinicians and support staff in improving interactions with their patients…I hope the next time I visit a conventional medical office or institution, the clinicians and support staff I meet have read this book."

British Columbia Naturopathic Association Bulletin

....

"An 'easy read' that I would recommend for both students and working PAs alike."

Maryland Association of Physicians Assistants

....

"With its emphasis on practical ways to show empathy, *Healing from the Heart* will truly help nurses increase levels of both patient and nursing satisfaction."

Loretta Turon, RN, MSN, MBA, CNA, Director Medical/Surgical, St. Joseph Medical Center (An ANCC Nursing Magnet)

"Direct care staffing is one of the greatest challenges for the healthcare profession. *Healing from the Heart* is an invaluable tool to address the many issues that contribute to staff turnover. This book will enable you to convey to your staff the empowerment they need. Without a doubt, this resource will make a lasting impact on your direct care workforce and ultimately, the quality of care and services of your organization."

Mary Brinkley, Executive Director, Oklahoma Association of Homes and Services for the Aging, El Reno, OK

....

"The concepts and exercises that Tim Dawes provides in *Healing from the Heart* will serve as a valuable resource to healthcare providers as they work to strengthen their communication with patients."

Pamela Popp, Senior Director, Office of Risk Management, Stanford University Medical Center, and Past President of the American Society for Healthcare Risk Management, Palo Alto, CA

....

"What an amazing tool! Easy to understand and very true to life. The coaching dialogues will help caregivers apply the skills back on the floor."

Maureen Mahoney, Director of Service Excellence, Childrens Memorial Hospital, Chicago, IL

....

"The central skill in empathy is the ability to uncover and meet needs, our patients' and our own. *Healing from the Heart* gives you a step-by-step process to do just that."

Kurt O'Brien, Organization Development Consultant, University of Washington Medical Center, Seattle, WA

....

"Cutting-edge health care recognizes the central role of the relationship between the caregiver and the patient. In *Healing from the Heart*, Tim Dawes gives medical staff a "how to" guide for nurturing that relationship."

Tammy Ream, Coordinator of Clinical Education, Texas Tech University Health Sciences Center PA Program, Midland, TX

"Empathy has benefits for providers as well as patients as it can reduce the stress of providers when they feel rushed or stressed by the demands of today's healthcare environment. Recognizing the patients' "experience" also allows the staff to understand and appreciate the psychological needs of the patient and address those needs in a compassionate way."

The Journal of Healthcare Risk Management

....

"Tim Dawes's workbooks avoid the pitfalls common to other manuals on patient service. Instead of merely instructing caregivers to parrot a patient's judgments, it gives them concrete ways to draw out patient needs that staffs can respond to."

Pam Kohles, Employee Health, Education, and Infection Control Coordinator, Lincoln Surgical Hospital. Lincoln, NE

....

"I like the approach in *Healing from the Heart*. It's almost as if Tim were with me coaching me through a live session."

Wally Leary, Director of Diversity, Erlanger Health System, Chattanooga, TN

....

"The NAHC puts a premium on the relationship between the family and caregiver. *Healing from the Heart* will be a useful tool to foster that relationship."

Mary St. Pierre, Vice President of Regulatory Affairs, Nat'l Assoc. for Home Care and Hospice, Washington, DC

....

"I see a lot of training material in my job. What strikes me about *Healing from the Heart* is the level of detail and the quality of the examples. The role plays will help put the skills into action."

Tulika Bhardawaj, Assistant Manager - Training, GE Healthcare, New Delhi, India

Healing from the Heart

A Practical Guide
to Creating Excellent Experiences
for Patients and Their Families

by
Timothy Dawes

Interplay Press, LLC
2829 W. Lk. Sammamish Pkwy SE
Bellevue, WA 98008
www.interplaygroup.com

Healing from the Heart...A Practical Guide to Creating Excellent Experiences for Patients and Their Families

A publication of Interplay Press, LLC.

Interplay Press, LLC. Permissions
2829 W. Lk. Sammamish Pkwy SE
Bellevue, WA 98008

Healing from the Heart...A Practical Guide to Creating Excellent Experiences for Patients and Their Families
First Edition, July 2006

Author: Timothy Dawes
Editor: Kaari Busick
Visual Design: Kimball Williams

Manufactured in the United States of America

We must become the change we want to see in the world.
Mohandas Gandhi

Contents

Preface

You're about to embark on a course designed to help you make your natural compassion visible to patients. You might wonder what the evidence and experts have to say about the effectiveness of empathy in treating patients.

You might also wonder about the place empathy skills occupy among your many initiatives—patient satisfaction, patient safety, quality improvement, and others.

While this is not an academic paper or policy manual, I'd like to give you an overview of what's been uncovered about the power of empathy in healthcare. I've also given you a brief bibliography of sources in the back in case you'd like to read more deeply.

The Case for Empathy Skills

There are at least four lines of evidence and reasoning for employing empathy with patients.

Skills that help you understand patients are likely to produce better treatment outcomes. Good treatment depends on meeting the patient's physical and emotional needs at the time they're under care, not some generalized notion of the needs of a class or category of patient (Bonder, 2001). You'll be most successful gathering culturally and clinically relevant information using qualitative methods. Qualitative strategies can provide meaningful insights about the interaction of the patient's culture with the current health situation (McClure and Teyber, 1996). The most effective methods emphasize empathy, intense listening, and curiosity (Rubin and Rubin, 1995).

Skills that help you listen to patients, and identify and satisfy their needs may lead to better health outcomes.

The central observation behind this line of reasoning is that patients who are more satisfied also show better compliance to treatment plans. Satisfied patients have improved medication compliance (Becker 1972), fewer missed appointments (Alpertgood, 1964), and improved overall compliance, at least in psychiatric patients (Eisenthal, 1979) and CHF patients (Hulka, 1976).

As you know, connecting treatment compliance to health outcomes is a complicated business. There is some positive evidence though. Improved patient satisfaction among diabetic patients, for example, has been correlated with better insulin compliance, fewer insulin reactions, and better perceived health status (Starfield, 1981).

The connection between patient satisfaction and empathy is clear, at least if you ask patients. A recent Harris Poll asked adults what they most wanted in a doctor. Their top four answers were indications of the doctor's empathy (treats you with dignity and respect, listens carefully to your health care concerns and questions, is easy to talk to, takes your concerns seriously). These factors scored higher than the doctor's medical training or medical judgment (Wall Street Journal, 2004). Look at the top three drivers of patient satisfaction in the largest study ever conducted and you'll find two of them (nurses anticipated your needs, and staff responded with care and compassion) measure the staff's ability to show empathy (Wolosin, 2003).

Empathy is therapeutic in and of itself. The feeling of being understood by another person bridges the "isolation of illness" (O'Neil, 1993). Empathy helps restore the sense of connectedness that patients need to feel whole (Suchman, 1998).

Finally, empathy decreases liability for your organization. The majority of your organization's malpractice suits don't spring from medical negligence (Mello and Hemenway,

2004). Patients sue because they don't like how they are being treated (Forster et al, 2002). They see themselves as deserted, think that their views are devalued, don't like the way information is reported to them, and believe that their physician doesn't understand their perspective (Beckman et al, 1994).

Lack of awareness about cultural differences may result in liability. Providers may discover that they are liable as a result of treatment in the absence of informed consent. Also, providers' or patients' failure to understand health beliefs, practices and behavior potentially constitutes a breach professional standards of care (National Center for Cultural Competency).

A 1994 study appearing in the journal of the American Medical Association showed that the ability to communicate well with patients is effective in reducing the likelihood of malpractice claims (NCCC). In fact, if your interest is in lowering liability, you may be better served by learning communications skills and showing patients you value their views than by decreasing actual rates of malpractice (Mello and Hemenway, 2004).

I'd add a fifth argument. I believe your experience of providing care to patients will improve with your ability to demonstrate the empathy you already feel. That conviction is a major driver for me in offering this guide to you.

The Place for Empathy Skills Among Your Strategic Initiatives

If your organization is like most, you have a number of initiatives going on already, including patient satisfaction, patient safety, quality improvement, and others. You may wonder where empathy skills fit in.

In some cases, empathy skills constitute an important part of the initiative itself. If you're running a residency program, for example, you may consider empathy at the intersection of communications, professionalism, and systems based practice.

In other cases, empathy skills will feed your initiatives. Empathy skills will help you learn more about your patients. That knowledge in turn will help you deliver better service. You'll notice opportunities to forge those connections as you go through the remainder of this material. And I'll call them out explicitly for you in the conclusion.

Acknowledgments

I would like to recognize the generosity of many people who critiqued this material and offered their suggestions for making it better. They include:

∴ Dr. Nancy Moore, Sr. Vice President Healing Health Services, Chief Nursing Officer, St. Charles Medical Center, Redmond, OR

∴ Dr. Paul O'Connor, Executive Director, Residency Review Committee for Obstetrics and Gynecology, the Accreditation Council for Graduate Medical Education (ACGME), Chicago, IL

∴ Michele Quirolo, President and CEO, VNA of Hudson Valley, Mt. Kisco, NY

∴ Mary St. Pierre, Vice President of Regulatory Affairs, the National Association of Home and Hospice Care (NAHC), Washington, DC

∴ Dr. Karen Drenkard, Chief Nurse Executive, Vice President Nursing, Inova Health System, Falls Church, VA

∴ Pamela Popp, Senior Director, Office of Risk Management, Past President, American Society for Healthcare Risk Management (ASHRM), Stanford University Medical Center, Palo Alto, CA

∴ Fay Rozovsky, President, The Rozovsky Group, Past President, American Society for Healthcare Risk Management (ASHRM), Bloomfield, CT

∴ Dr. Barry Egener, Medical Director, The Foundation For Medical Excellence (TFME), Portland, OR

∴ Wally Leary, Director of Diversity, Erlanger Health System, Chattanooga, TN

∴ Maureen Mahoney, Director of Service Excellence, Childrens Memorial Hospital, Chicago, IL

∴ Loretta Turon, Medical Surgical Director, St. Joseph Medical Center Paterson, NJ

∴ Kurt O'Brien, Organization Development Consultant, Organization Development and Training, University of Washington Medical Center, Seattle, WA

∴ Pam Kohles, Employee Health and Education Coordinator, Lincoln Surgery Hospital, Lincoln, NB

∴ Tammy Ream, Coordinator of Clinical Education, TTUHSC PA Program, Midland, TX

∴ Jan Haedt, Sr. Risk Management Consultant, University of Wisconsin Hospital and Clinics, Madison, WI

∴ Jennifer Woodburn, St. Camillus Health and Rehabilitation Center, Syracuse, NY

∴ Tulika Bhardawaj, Assistant Manager—Training, GE Healthcare, New Delhi, India

∴ Bobbie Bagley, BDB Health Promotions, Hudson, NH

I'm grateful to have been able to work with so many gifted trainers in developing this work. Wes Taylor, a partner at the NVC Training Institute and counselor specializing in addictions and trauma survivors, helped to create and teach the original curriculum. Along the way, I've co-taught the course with a large number of talented trainers including, Melanie Sears, a veteran nurse who has been using NVC in healthcare for over a dozen years, Kathleen Macferran, Holly Eckert, Liv Monroe, Doug Dolstad, Barbara Larson, and Jerry Jaz.

I'm grateful also to Dr. Jim Boggs, my original mentor who started me in this work and taught me the importance of honoring trainees and making training an act of service.

And finally, my deep appreciation goes to Caron MacLane and Sabina Nawaz both talented independent trainers and consultants in Seattle, Washington who have supported me in every aspect of my work for years, and especially to my wife, Lisa Phelps Dawes, who is my partner in every venture.

Of course, the final decisions concerning what goes between these covers and what does not are mine alone.

Disclaimer

This workbook is designed to help caregivers develop their ability to make their natural compassion visible to patients. The publisher and author aren't engaged in rendering legal advice or service, risk management, or other professional services. If you or your staff requires risk management, legal assistance, or other expert assistance, please seek the services of a competent professional on your staff or in your community.

Caregivers work in a very complex environment for communications. As you apply the skills you learn here, you'll need to take into account a variety of factors that influence and constrain what you can say. These include HIPAA requirements, patients and staff members who come from other cultures and speak other languages, patient safety, process improvement, and risk management projects and guidelines, core competencies demanded by organizations such as the ACGME and others, your own sense of safety in the midst of others who may be angry or mean you harm, and more.

This workbook doesn't contain all the available information about communicating with patients and staff members. My intention is to complement, amplify, and supplement other crucial material you have access to. For examples, contact Risk Management, Human Resources, or representatives of similar functions in your medical group. I urge you to read all the available material, learn as much as possible about sound interpersonal communications and the rules, laws, and guidelines that apply to you, and tailor the information in this workbook to your work environment.

The purpose of this manual is to provide staffs with insights and skills that others have found useful. Staffs use this material at their own discretion. The author and Interplay shall have neither liability nor responsibility to any person or entity with respect to any loss or damage caused, or alleged to have been caused, directly or indirectly, by the information or recommendations contained in this workbook.

If you do not wish to be bound by the above, you may return this book to the publisher for a full refund.

Making Your Empathy Visible to Patients

Of course, you're already compassionate. You made that clear when you chose healthcare as your field. You prove it every day in the level of care you provide, the effort you put in, and the things you do to help people and make them comfortable. And you're already a healer, a skillful one.

So why pick up a workbook that offers to teach you empathy skills for healers?

This workbook will help you create more of what you wanted when you turned to healing as a profession.

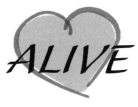

Assess your
   rapport

Listen for a call
   for help

Intend to
   connect

Verify what's
   alive

Encourage a
   request that
   enriches life

More of what you're looking for...

You'd like better outcomes for your patients. You want to heal people. Empathy skills will help you do that. When people receive empathy, they feel honored. And when they feel honored, they're more open, freer to reveal the kind of personal information that will help you provide better care.

And the benefits flow both ways. Here's what I mean.

Think of something concrete you've done recently that made life better for someone. Could be anyone—a patient, another caregiver, your spouse, your kids, a stranger. How do you feel when you think of that?

Proud…fulfilled…happy…even powerful?

That's remarkable when you think about it—that you feel so filled up from having given to someone else.

A gift of the heart benefits both the giver and the receiver. When you receive empathy, you get the gift of being seen and understood with no expectations or obligations attached. And when you give empathy, you feel the thrill of contribution.

And isn't that why you became a healer—to feel the joy and self-esteem that come from contributing to others?

When you find it tough to create the experiences you're seeking

As a healer, you have a full store of gifts to offer your patients. You diagnose their ills, prescribe treatments, carry out procedures, assess progress, and dispense advice and medication.

"Empathy supplements objective knowledge, and the use of technology, and other tools for making accurate diagnoses."

Bioethicist
Jody Halpern

Most of the time, you have just what your patients need.

But there are difficult times as well, aren't there? You give of yourself and your patients don't seem responsive to you.

What's the difference between patient encounters that go well and those that don't?

That's the question I've focused on for the past several years. While you handle most interactions with grace, why is it that others seem challenging? What makes some encounters with people, patients in particular, difficult? Why do you enjoy some encounters with patients while others leave you frustrated?

I had an opportunity to explore questions like those in my work in an innovative program carried out in one of the largest universities in the country. Over the course of 6 years, the project produced over 500 education and training programs.

I was particularly drawn to the training we provided for face-to-face interactions using "standardized" scenarios—people coached to simulate an actual sufferer (victim,

2

patient, or family member) so accurately that the simulation seems real to experts and the people being trained.

Among those training sessions, we noticed a very important pattern.

In a group of journalists interviewing victims of an apartment fire, for example, one reporter came away with a list of details for a story while another, interviewing the same person, grumbled that the witness was unapproachable.

In a group of respiratory therapists assessing a woman with Chronic Obstructive Pulmonary Disorder, one therapist came away disheartened and angry while another actually laughed through the assessment.

We saw it again and again, whether we were working with neo-natal nurses, nurses assessing developmental loss, therapists, organ donor coordinators, AIDS volunteers, or medical caseworkers.

One caregiver would walk away from a sufferer feeling satisfied and successful, even joyful. Another would leave the same sufferer feeling angry and stifled, having made little headway.

As we looked closely at the interactions that seemed most successful, we recognized some similarities.

∴ In the most successful encounters, the caregiver focused his attention in a particular way.

∴ The comfort and experience of the sufferers became an important element of the interaction.

∴ That shift in focus led the caregivers in effective encounters to ask different questions and make different suggestions than those in ineffective encounters who got stuck somehow simply "doing their jobs."

A way to turn your best instincts into deliberate actions

"In the encounters that were most successful, caregivers found a way to create rapport with their patients."

In the encounters that were most successful, caregivers found a way to create rapport with their patients. That probably doesn't surprise you. That's how you operate most of the time. But when we're not conscious about how we create rapport, the ability can escape us when we need it most.

So, I set out to find a skill set that would help frontline caregivers create connections with their patients—dependably and reliably—even when patients are most difficult to reach.

That's what you'll find in these workbooks, the ALIVE model of empathy—**a framework for expressing yourself honestly and clearly, that makes your respect and compassion visible to patients**.

It's based on the work of Marshall Rosenberg and the Center for Nonviolent Communication, www.cnvc.org (and a portion of the proceeds from this material goes to his organization). NVC is a system that focuses on fostering connection and negotiating strategies for action. I've adapted NVC for the particular demands of healthcare.

By fostering deep understanding between you and your patient, this model helps you create the connection you're looking for—a connection based on the joy of giving to one another from the heart.

4

This isn't new information. It's a way of organizing what you already know and what you already do when you're most effective, so that you get the experience you're looking for and the results you want more consistently.

What Active Empathy Is And What It Will Do For You

You probably have your own idea of what empathy is. For the purposes of this training, we'll define empathy skills rigorously. In particular, we'll focus on skills that will enable you to create the kind of experiences you and your patients value most.

Let's look at those kinds of experiences. Here are three examples of encounters that have left patients very satisfied and feeling closer to a caregiver:

∴ My cough made me scream. A nurse appeared from nowhere and pushed at my side to keep my inflamed lung from pressing at my ribs.

∴ I was admitted to inpatient psych. I'd wake up angry. Somehow, the therapists were able to listen to and talk with me without treating me as poorly as I treated them.

∴ I was in bed crying as I was recovering from a procedure. A nurse arrived with my sleeping pill, turned off the light, and held my hand until I had cried myself out

Your Turn

Think of two encounters you've had with healthcare organizations that have been so powerful they left lasting impressions. Try to think of one experience in which you were the patient (someone may have stopped what they were doing to attend to you) and one in which you were the caregiver (you might, for example, have said something that put a fearful patient at ease).

"The research evidence has kept piling up, and it points strongly to the conclusion that a high degree of empathy in a relationship is possibly the most potent factor in bringing about change and learning."

Carl Rogers,
A Way of Being

My encounter as a patient:

_____

_____

_____

My encounter as a caregiver:

_____

_____

_____

What specifically did you do or experience that made the encounter so memorable for you?

For example, Shauna felt she had irregular heartbeats, and nausea. Her doctor took some tests that turned out negative. When Shauna said she was still concerned her doctor offered to have her assistant check Shauna's medications. They found she was taking a medication which had been recalled because it caused symptoms like hers.

What I experienced as a patient:

_____

_____

_____

_____

_____

What I did or experienced as a caregiver:

_____

_____

_____

_____

_____

_____

As you reflect on your own experiences as a patient and as a caregiver, what do you see as the common elements of memorable experiences in medical care?

What I find makes encounters memorable and satisfying as a patient (and caregiver):

empathy
[ém·pə·thee],
noun, _a respectful understanding of another person's reality_

_____

_____

_____

_____

_____

Many lists will include elements like these:

∴ My caregiver listened to me

∴ My caregiver took me seriously

∴ My caregiver understood what I needed

∴ My caregiver anticipated my concerns or responded to me in a way that met my needs

In fact, elements like these rank at the top of most lists of keys to patient satisfaction and loyalty. They're really just a summary of what many of us would want in any encounter that's respectful and nurturing. And we'll turn to this list to define empathy skills.

For the purpose of this program, we'll define them this way:

Empathy skills support healers in creating heartfelt connections with patients—so each has the experience of being listened to respectfully and having their needs taken seriously.

"The challenge is not to become more compassionate, but to find ways to strengthen your natural compassion and make it more visible to patients, even in times of stress."

The ALIVE model will aid you in creating heart-to-heart connections with your patients (and anyone else in your life). The hallmark of these connections is sincere mutuality, an encounter in which you and others feel deeply heard and respected.

There are a couple of important things to notice about this definition of empathy skills:

∴ This isn't a "patient is always right" program. In fact, this perspective is an alternative to making patients right, or wrong. The ALIVE model calls us to **be curious about the experience our patient is having, rather than label him or her in any way**.

∴ This is not a "whatever the patient wants" program. We emphasize mutual respect. We'll suggest a framework for satisfying patient requests. But the goal of that framework is to help you **meet everyone's needs—yours, your patient's, and your organization's**.

10

Empathy skills and patient care

You're a healer. But what does that mean? Certainly, your patients and your organization look to you to as part of a team that diagnoses and treats the sick.

But there's more isn't there? You have a part in providing patient service. Even maintaining patient satisfaction.

Empathy Skills
What's in it for you?

1. You'll have less stress because fewer confrontations will escalate

2. You'll feel more confident

3. You'll be more likely to get what you're seeking because patients and others will hear your compassion

4. You'll create deeper connections with patients with less risk

5. You'll be more effective at putting cultural awareness information into practice

6. You'll have more of the healing experiences that attracted you to healthcare in the first place

No doubt, you'll think of many more.

What role does empathy play in all that? Empathy faces you with a bit of a paradox. On one hand, you mean to fill everything you do with compassion. On the other, you may despair of finding the time to show empathy to even one patient in the degree you'd like. There is a way to resolve this seeming paradox.

Al Stubblefield, CEO of Baptist Health Care, tells the story of how his hospital handled a nagging patient service issue. "Staff's concern for your privacy" ranked among the top complaints from patients of Baptist Health Care, as it did for patients throughout the industry.

His staff closed the door when entering a patient's room, and drew the curtain before they began a procedure.

And still their patients registered lack of concern for privacy as a major complaint. Finally, they taught their staff to mention the steps they were taking and to tie those actions to the patient's needs. "I've closed the door and pulled the curtain because I want you to feel comfortable. Do you have the privacy you need?"

As a complaint, "staff's concern for privacy" fell near the bottom of the list at Baptist Health Care, as it did for other hospitals who instituted similar scripts.

Did the staff suddenly become more concerned for patients? No. They were concerned all along. **What changed was their ability to communicate their concern in ways patients could see.**

Scripts like these are effective tools once you've discovered a common need. This workbook program will help you in ways scripts can't.

This program will help you create great experiences for yourself and your patients

It will:

∴ teach you a process you can use in patient interactions that's as flexible as you are and as fluid as the interactions you encounter every day,

∴ help you focus your attention in a way that maintains your compassion even when you're facing great stress,

∴ help you uncover patient needs quickly.

We've seen some surprising results from making compassion more visible to patients.

∴ **Encounters often take less time than you expect**. Nothing is faster than an efficient staff person working with an agreeable patient. Very often though, the resistance patients put up slows things down. A demonstration of your sincere compassion will often create the safety patients need to release that resistance.

∴ **Patients seem more manageable**. Caregivers have told us that patients who once appeared to them as curt and rude, emotionally unstable, even "unreachable" show up as people with specific reasons to have deep fears, sorrow, or fatigue, once the staff becomes deliberate about demonstrating their own compassion more clearly.

∴ **You'll feel stronger as you teach yourself to expect respect from others.** When we're brusque, we come to believe we live in a rude world. As you make your compassion more visible to others, you'll show yourself that other people could be considerate of you, even when you make mistakes. The more you offer compassion, the more you'll come to expect it from others.

Not-So Close Encounters

We all have a variety of strategies we use to connect with each other. You may use them with your patients. Think how often you've said or heard something like this.

Strategy	What you might have said or overheard
Advising	"You should really ask Dr. Anderson about this, because…"
Easing	"If you think you're in bad shape, you should see the boy down the hall."
Educating	"Oh, this is very common. What we usually see next is…" or "We have this policy in order to keep patients safe."
Consoling	"It wasn't your fault. It's the disease process."
Encouraging	"You've got to be strong for your family. You can do this."
Telling Stories	"I remember once we had a man in here who…"
Sympathizing	"Oh, you poor thing…"
Interrogating/ Diagnosing	"When did you first notice this?" or "Where exactly to you feel the pain?"

These strategies often work. We resort to them almost unconsciously. The great strength of these strategies is that they move the action forward quickly. They're shorthand. If you were to speak your entire thought out loud, it might sound something like this.

∴ **"You're confused** about your treatment plan**? You need information** or a referral for where you can get it. You should really **ask Dr. Anderson…"**

∴ **"You're feeling guilty** about the part you believe you played in your husband's illness? **You need consolation.** I'd like you to know that **it wasn't your fault."**

∴ "You think your case is so bad you can't be helped. **You're scared. You need reassurance. Let me tell you** about a man I saw last month…"

The great strength of these strategies is also their great weakness. By moving the action forward, they can leave the patient thinking they've been bypassed. The strategies backfire when your patient wants someone to **acknowledge their unique experience**, when his trust in you or your organization is being tested, or when she simply needs to be seen or heard as an individual.

That's why we suggest you use empathy of the kind we're describing.

To remind yourself of what it's like for someone to hear these strategies when they want some different response, imagine yourself as the mother in the scenario below from a unit we worked with in a large hospital.

As you read the nurse's responses, write down your gut reaction in the spaces I've provided. (There is no right or wrong reaction. Your reaction is true for you.) I've put the strategies in [brackets] to make them easy to identify.

You are a 28 year old Eastern European immigrant, and a mother of three. You clean houses in a small rural town to support your family.

Three months ago, your son Anton began to complain of stomach pain. You didn't take him seriously. When he persisted, you set up an appointment with your doctor. It was nine days before you had a day off to take him in. By that time, he had been throwing up for three days and showing bruises you couldn't account for.

Your doctor suspected cancer and put you and your son on a bus to the nearest large hospital. Three days later, a hematologist in the hospital confirmed that Anton had leukemia.

Currently, he's on the 7th week of a repeating protocol of chemotherapy and rest. His white cell count has fallen almost to zero. He's vomiting with frequent headaches. Yesterday, his doctor recommended that you put Anton on a ventilator.

A nurse enters Anton's room, responding to your call button.

Nurse: Hi, I'm Nancy. I'll be Anton's nurse tonight. Is everything all right? I saw the call button.

Mother: (in a heavy accent, and very haltingly) You make, ah…prayer with me?

Nurse: You want to pray? Oh. Yes. I can get you someone from Pastoral Care [problem solving].

Mother: No. You…please. Sit. Please…talk.

Nurse: It's OK. You're Eastern Orthodox, aren't you? I'm sure we have a chaplain who [recommending]…

Mother: No…please. Please. It is…my fault.

Nurse: What? Your fault? No, it's not your fault [consoling]. Look, I'm sorry, I don't…Why don't I get you a translator?

Mother: No! My fault. Anton is… leukemia. My fault. Nine days. Too long.

Nurse: No, no. It's not your fault [consoling, again]. Leukemia is a blood disease [educating]. It's nobody's fault.

How you feel inside as the mother hearing this response:

_____

_____

_____

Mother: Yes, yes, my fault. God is…punish me (she starts to cry). I bad. No good. No money.

Nurse: No, no. You're a good mother. You've done everything you can [encouraging]. Why don't you let me… Can I get you a drink of water? Why don't I get you a drink of water [problem solving]?

How you feel inside as the mother hearing this response:

_____

_____

_____

Mother: No, no. You say…what I do. Doctor say…ventilator. (tears come to her eyes).

Nurse: A ventilator? Oh, you should really talk to your doctor about that [advising]. Let me get him for you, all right?

How you feel inside as the mother hearing this response:

_____

_____

_____

Mother: No. No. You. What you do?

Nurse: Oh, I can't tell you what to do. You're his mother. You know him better than anyone. You'll know the right thing to do [encouraging].

_____

_____

_____

You've been exploring your own reactions to some ways people habitually respond to patients in grief. Your reactions may be unique to you. We've run this scenario for hundreds of frontline medical staff and administrative managers. I can tell you what they report after seeing it.

They view the nurse as rushed despite the time she spends with the mother. And they see her as uncaring and a poor listener despite the variety of solutions she proposes in response to the mother's pleas.

But the nurse isn't uncaring. When we debriefed a nurse following an encounter like this, she said she wanted to cry and didn't know why. It's likely because she desperately wanted to help the mother and ended up acutely frustrated.

It's conversations like these, when you can't find a way to connect and contribute, that burn you out. They cause "stress hangovers" that last for days.

There's nothing wrong with the nurse or the strategies she chose. She used them because they often work for her. They just weren't responsive for this patient.

You likely recognized a number of opportunities for the nurse to change the tenor of the encounter by acknowledging the mother's predicament.

∴ "You sound as though you feel terribly guilty."

∴ "You're desperate to be sure Anton is getting the best possible care."

∴ "You want so much to know you're making a good decision."

It's what we'd all say on our good days.

This encounter was tough for this nurse on this day. What the nurse needs is a way of reminding herself how to connect with her patient when other strategies fail, when she's confronting a person who's challenging for her, or when she's having a difficult day.

An Introduction to the ALIVE Model of Empathy

What do you do when you sense that the strategies that normally help you connect with your patients fail to work?

I recommend you use active empathy—a deliberate way of interacting that makes your compassion more visible to patients. Especially patients in distress.

Out of our training work, we've developed a model of active empathy that many caregivers have found helpful. The process is called the ALIVE model of empathy and it's comprised of these steps:

Assess your rapport

Listen for a call for help

Intend to connect

Verify what's alive

Encourage a request that enriches life

The ALIVE model focuses us on honesty, clarity, and connection. It alerts us to opportunities to connect with patients in ways that are more effective and more satisfying.

As we focus on connecting, and on clarifying what we and our patients feel and need, rather than on blaming, labeling, or fixing each other, we continually rediscover our common humanity and the depth of our compassion.

The respect and empathy that follows from this conscious connection fosters a mutual desire to give to each other from the heart.

Assess your rapport

Listen for a call for help

Intend to connect

Verify what's alive

Encourage a request that enriches life

A note before we get started

You're looking at a model for connecting with patients that's composed of five steps and covered in a workbook 150 pages long. That might seem a bit intimidating at first.

You may take some comfort in knowing that ALIVE doesn't represent a whole new way of communicating. Don't expect to find a lot of new concepts on the following pages or descriptions of lengthy procedures to follow.

Rather, what you'll encounter is a series of insights and distinctions. It's a systematic way of thinking about what you've been doing well all along, so you can create the outcomes you value more consistently.

"You do this already in many circumstances. The challenge is to seize opportunities for connection no matter how they show up."

The first three steps in the ALIVE model—Assess your rapport, Listen for a call for help, and Intend to connect—are largely shifts in attitude. They set the stage for creating strong connections.

The fourth step—Verify what's alive—is the actual process of connecting with the patient. The fifth step—Encourage a request—is when you generate strategies that meet your needs as well as the needs of your patient and your healthcare organization.

Putting the model into practice doesn't have to take long or be laborious.

Imagine, for example, you walk into a patient's room to deliver a sedative. You see tears on her cheeks only briefly as she turns her face from you. Guessing that she's fearful about an impending surgery, you decide not to talk. Instead, you turn out the lights, take a seat close by, and set your hand on the bed in case she wants to take it.

You've just accomplished the entire model in the matter of a few heartbeats. And without saying a word.

You do this already in many circumstances. The challenge is to seize opportunities for connection no matter how they show up—whether your patient is weeping in bed, threatening to sue, swearing at you, or asking you what he should tell his son about God.

That's what this program will help you do.

In this Unit, we'll take a brief look at each step in the model. In the next Section of the workbook, you'll get lots of examples and opportunities for practice.

Signs that you don't have high-quality rapport with your patient

1. You don't sense an easy flow

2. You're afraid to say what you mean or what you feel

3. You're not breathing easily

4. You feel an uncomfortable tension in your body

5. You're having an experience of life that you wouldn't choose

Other signs you notice:

6. _____

_____

_____

7. _____

_____

_____

Assess your rapport

As part of our training programs, I sometimes ask caregivers when they think it would be a good time to give empathy. Inevitably, I hear, "once you have rapport". My experience is just the opposite. Giving empathy is an effective way to connect with your patient or reestablish the connection once you've lost it.

How do you know when you've lost rapport?

You can assess your rapport by paying attention to what *you* are experiencing. Not your feelings—your happiness, sadness, fear, or anger—but your sense of openness and ease in your communication with your patient. You know from experience that you can sense tension in the air when people aren't connected.

Think of an interaction in which you've had an easy flow back and forth. Even if it was a tough topic, you were able to speak frankly. You felt the other person heard you and you heard them. Any time you don't feel that easy flow, you don't have rapport.

All of the signs listed in the box on the previous page are signals of resistance. Each is a reason to give empathy.

Listen for a call for help

Quit Taking It Personally (QTIP). That's a common admonition in customer service these days. When your customer or patient gets upset, don't take it personally. What you don't hear is how to take it, if not personally.

ALIVE reminds us to take our patients' statements not as a comment about us but as a sign of their needs or their suffering.

By focusing your attention this way, you'll hear any comment directed at you as the best strategy your patient could find to get some need met.

Some statements are obvious calls for help:

∴ "I need some privacy."

∴ "Would you explain this to me?"

∴ "Can you make me more comfortable?"

We recognize immediately that we're being called to action. If we're left with a question, it's only how to act most effectively.

rapport [ra·páwr], noun, *an easy relationship people enjoy based on mutual trust, and a sense that they understand each other's concerns.*

24

Some statements patients make aren't so obviously calls for help. They're dressed in a language of judgment, blame, or threat.

∴ "How can you tell me to stop treatment?"

∴ "We both know what's going on here. Do I even need to say it?"

∴ "You try to stop me and I'll sue this office and I'll sue you, too."

∴ "You know what you are? A racist, plain and simple!"

Statements like these may not sound like a call for help. But my experience with patients and caregivers is that **we are always either asking for help or showing gratitude.**

"That's what your patients want. Not a bad experience for you but a better experience for them."

For example:

∴ A son who asks, "How can you tell me to stop treatment for my mother?" may be telling you **he needs to know he can trust** your judgment, or he needs to figure out how he can think of himself as a good son.

∴ A woman who says, "You try to stop me and I'll sue this office and I'll sue you, too" may be telling you **she needs to know she has some say** in how her life goes.

∴ A man who calls you a racist may be telling you **he wants the same respect** anyone else receives.

None of these points will be great revelations to you. Each is just a simple shift in perspective. Think about it. There's little payoff for a patient to brow beat you into admitting, for instance, that you're inept. But there's a great payoff for that patient to enlist you in ensuring she gets responsible care.

That's what your patients want. Not a bad experience for you but a better experience for them.

A supervising nurse I worked with recently told me, "I'm not a racist, but there's nothing I can say to change this patient's mind." That's the core. If you hear a judgment about you, you'll try to defend yourself. Nothing you can say will be enough.

Shift your perspective. See your patient as suffering and calling for help. And you'll open up a whole new line of responses.

Intend to connect

In short, **Get Curious**. If you're not coming from curiosity, you're not in a position to give empathy.

You can certainly create connection without empathy. In the previous Unit, we covered a list of strategies people often use to create connection.

But when those strategies fail you, you need to become curious about whatever it is your patient is going through.

When we don't form a conscious intention like being curious, most of us will unconsciously try to fix patients or get them to do what we want. It's how we've been brought up.

If your intention is to fix your patients, they'll pick up on it. No matter the words you choose, your patients won't like it. And they'll let you know.

Here's an example:

A medical case-worker talks with a mother who is terribly frightened.

26

Caseworker: "OK, I get that you're upset. And you want to get out of here. And I want to help you. But you've got to fill out this paperwork before you can take your daughter home."

Mother: "I don't want to hear all this institutional talk. You leave me alone. I'll sue if I have to!"

The case-worker identified how the mother is feeling and what she wants. So why isn't she grateful?

Because his intention is to get her to take some action he's already decided on, not to connect with her or be curious about her.

"The capacity to give one's attention to a sufferer is a very rare and difficult thing; it is almost a miracle; it is a miracle."

Simone Weil

In fact, when I asked him what he thought the mother was going through, he said he was so busy trying to get her to do what he wanted and make her think it was her idea that he wasn't paying attention to how she was feeling.

She could tell.

I don't suggest that you abandon your agenda whenever you enter a patient's room. I do suggest that when your patient puts up resistance, you bracket your agenda, trust yourself to come back to it, and find out what experience your patient is having—as an end in itself.

What might that look like?

Notice in the example above, the caseworker's agenda is to get the mother to fill out the paperwork. If he brackets that agenda, his goal will be simply to find out what's behind the mother's actions.

He might ask, for example:

Caseworker: "Are you afraid for your daughter for some reason?"

The mother may or may not be. If she's not, the caseworker can ask more questions. In the Units that follow, we'll suggest ways to formulate those questions so you make quick and effective progress.

Notice that the first three steps of the ALIVE model can be done in seconds or less. It's a quick internal check followed by a couple of shifts in perspective—Assess your rapport, Listen for a call for help, Intend to connect. Together they prepare you mentally to engage effectively with your patient.

Verify what's alive

Recall that we make these shifts in thinking to prepare the ground for a mutual desire to give from the heart.

And we nurture this mutual desire by focusing our attention on what's alive for our patient. In other words, what our patient is feeling and what she needs right now in this moment. That's a three-step process.

1. Observe what's happening. What are people saying or doing that's meeting your patient's needs or not meeting them? The trick that we'll explore in more depth is how to separate our judgments from our observations, how to simply describe actions.

2. Ask or suggest how your patient may be feeling when she observes those actions. Is she in pain, or afraid, irritated, or joyful?

3. Suggest which of your patient's needs might be behind their feelings. Does he need some relief, a better understanding of what's happening to his body, or some consideration for what he's going through?

We'll go through each of these steps in detail in Section Two.

For now, you might demonstrate your empathy to your patient by saying, "Felicia, are you apprehensive about being discharged because you need to know that you're ready for whatever comes next?"

Encourage a request to enrich life

The final step is to encourage your patient to make a request that would meet her needs.

For example, "Would it help for you to talk to someone about gathering a network of support around you?"

The dance of compassion

This is one side of the ALIVE model, seeking to understand these four aspects of your patients' experience.

The other side consists of expressing the same four aspects of your experience clearly. You connect by revealing what you observe, feel, and need, and the actions that would better meet your needs and the needs of your organization.

Together, the two sides form a kind of dance that you are likely already familiar with. As we attend to what is alive in our patients and express what is alive in ourselves, back and forth, we uncover our humanity.

What arises is a mutual desire to give from the heart.

We'll explore this model in greater depth in the next Section beginning with listening skills.

Although I'll give you a formula for creating clarity, it's important to remember that **the process itself isn't formulaic. You'll be adapting it to your personal style.**

I'd also like you to remember that while I'll be presenting you with some basic words to say, **talking is optional.**

29

When you give empathy to a grieving person for example, you can focus your attention with an internal dialogue as easily as talking. You can open yourself to all four aspects of your patient's experience without saying a single word out loud.

Make it Last

You are the key to lasting change

A core tenet of the ALIVE model is that **anything anyone does, he does in order to meet a need**.

That insight is crucial for you in dealing with patients, and critical for you in working with these skills.

You'll use these skills and deepen them over time; precisely to the extent that they help you meet your needs over time.

As you explore and work through these workbooks you'll have an opportunity to get clear about what you need and how you can gather support to get those needs met.

The Three Levers of Lasting Change

You have three levers that affect your ability to create lasting change in your life: *your beliefs, your practices, the environment of support you create.* Let's take a look at how these three interact to determine your success in creating change that lasts.

Arthur and Bethany

Imagine you have two patients, Arthur and Bethany, each trying to lose weight. You've counseled each to cut back on calories and increase their exercise.

Arthur believes he's big-boned and destined by heredity to gain and keep weight. He also thinks that exercise and weight loss is for women and younger kids and it's unbecoming for him.

Still, he makes a mental note to himself to cut back on eating. He's not inspired enough to count his calories or watch the glycemic index of the food he eats.

"You'll use these skills and deepen them over time; precisely to the extent that they help you meet your needs over time."

31

In the evenings, he often finds himself tempted to eat more while he's watching TV. And sometimes he thinks he can afford to because he doesn't recall eating a lot of fat or sugar during the day.

He goes to the gym three times a week and moves from machine to machine over the course of 45 minutes, taking short breaks when he's tired or uncomfortable.

Bethany, on the other hand, believes that the structures you're encouraging her to create can help her succeed. She climbed Mt. Rainier once when her friends thought she couldn't. She believes there are times when she can do the unexpected if she wants it enough.

> **Three Levers of Lasting Change**
>
> 1. Your beliefs
> 2. Your personal practices
> 3. A supportive environment

She puts together a chart of her starting weight and goal weight and creates a routine of weighing herself every morning at the same time. In fact, she buys a new scale that also reports her percentage body fat.

She buys a copy of Prevention Magazine, reads it cover to cover, and takes out a subscription. She clips pictures of women of her body type around her ideal weight and tapes them up around her mirror and on her refrigerator.

She tells two best friends that she's committed to losing weight, enlists one as a workout partner, and commits to sending a copy of her daily food intake to the other each night.

Who do you suppose will have the greatest motivation to continue his or her program?

It's a rhetorical question, isn't it? Bethany is changing her lifestyle. She's taking action to change her environment to support her goals. And she's drawing a community of support around her. Those actions create lasting change.

How about you?

The Three Levers of Lasting Change are at work in your life and your organization, right now. They're moving you in a direction, or holding you in place.

The first step is for you to become aware of the levers at work in your life. Take a few minutes and brainstorm about your beliefs, your practices, and your environment. How are you set up to get your needs met?

Beliefs

> *"Never doubt that a small group of thoughtful, committed citizens can change the world. Indeed, it is the only thing that ever has."*
>
> Margaret Mead

You'll notice that there are two kinds of beliefs. Boosters, the beliefs that tend to support you in reaching your goals. And Breakers, the beliefs that stand in your way. As far as weight loss is concerned, Arthur is heavy on Breakers. He thinks he has the kind of body that tends to pack on weight and that weight loss is for other people but not for him. Bethany, on the other hand, has developed a number of Boosters. Although she's struggled with weight, she's accomplished other goals and believes she has a reservoir of strength other people often miss. And she believes in the structures you've put together with her.

Your beliefs

What beliefs do you have that stand in your way (Breaker Beliefs)?

My Breaker Beliefs

1. _____

2. _____

3. _____

4. _____

5. _____

_____

_____

What beliefs do you have that support you (Booster Beliefs) in creating powerful interactions with patients?

My Booster Beliefs

1. _____

2. _____

3. _____

4. _____

5. _____

_____

_____

Personal practices

You saw a number of practices that either worked for or against the goal of weight loss. They included tracking progress or not. Watching TV or working out. Gathering a community of friends or going it alone.

Look at how you handle interactions with people today. What do you notice that helps you create powerful interactions or undermines you?

Here are some questions to ask yourself.

When I recall handling the difficult interactions in my life, how do I picture myself and what do I say about myself?

_____

_____

_____

_____

What do I read or watch on TV that influences how I interact with people?

_____

_____

_____

_____

What's the tenor of the informal "water cooler" conversations I have with people about work and interactions?

_____

_____

_____

_____

_____

Organizational Environment

We often underestimate the impact of our environment on our behavior and practices. There's a theory, for example, that a primary stimulus for the crime wave that hit New York City in the 80's was the number of broken windows that went unfixed in key neighborhoods. The broken windows sent a message that the neighbors didn't put much stock in the condition of the neighborhoods. They gave the impression that the City was a place where crime and neglect happen freely. And in fact, when the police cracked down on petty crime, crimes that are more serious began to plummet.

"It is possible to be a better person on a clean street or in a clean subway than in one littered with trash and graffiti."

Malcolm Gladwell

When I interview medical staff, they often name two to three policies their organization enforces that tend to incite conflict—no or low-tolerance for loud or abusive language, restrictive visitation policies, and the like. The policies can send a message that order is more important than patient experience.

Think about your organization and the environment you create for patients. What do you notice that helps you create powerful interactions or undermines you?

Here are some suggestions of things to think about.

Which of our policies or strategies tend to invite conflict with patients and how would we change them to be supportive instead?

_____

_____

_____

_____

How would we modify our signage or décor to send a message of support to our patients?

_____

_____

_____

_____

When we address patient concerns in internal meetings, what kinds of issues do we spotlight? And what is our predominant attitude?

_____

_____

_____

_____

Focus on empathy

This may seem like a lot to think about. You can give yourself a running start by thinking of a couple of things you can do in the next few days to keep "visible empathy" on your radar screen. Here are some suggestions we like:

∴ Arrange a weekly coffee with someone else who is working through this workbook, so you can compare notes.

∴ Get an agenda item on your next group meeting to talk about the environment you've created for patients and how supportive it is.

Things I can do to focus on empathy

1. _____

   _____

2. _____

   _____

3. _____

   _____

4. _____

   _____

5. _____

   _____

Listening with Empathy

In Section One, we defined empathy as a respectful understanding of another person's reality. And we described the goal for empathy skills:

∴ enable healers to create a connection with patients and their family members such that each has the experience of being listened to respectfully and having their needs taken seriously.

We described the ways you and your patients will benefit as you sharpen your empathy skills.

Patients:

∴ have better experiences,

∴ see themselves as better understood, and

∴ may even have better medical outcomes.

Care givers we've trained have also reported that

∴ interactions with patients—especially the ones they've considered tough—are more fulfilling,

∴ they are able to identify workable solutions to patient problems more quickly , and

∴ they have more of the experiences that drew them to healing in the first place.

You read about some of the habitual strategies for communicating we all use. And you explored your own reactions to hearing those strategies when you're hoping for a deeper connection with the speaker.

Finally, we introduced a process for demonstrating empathy that we've found useful for caregivers, the ALIVE model.

And we briefly described the five steps:

Assess your rapport

Listen for a call for help

Intend to connect

Verify what's alive

Encourage a request that enriches life

The first three steps—assess your rapport, listen for a call for help, and intend to connect—lay the groundwork for a powerful connection with patients. They can all be done literally in seconds.

The final two steps—verify what's alive and encourage a request that enriches life—encapsulate the process of interacting with patients to uncover needs and agree on solutions. We'll take up that process in more depth in this Section.

I See What You Mean

Clarifying the OBSERVATIONS you hear from your patients

The first step in the process of uncovering your patients' needs is to get clear about what they're seeing, hearing, and sensing that affects their well-being. **These are the kinds of things you can impact.**

One of the strongest habits we have as human beings is our tendency to judge things as we experience them. Almost in one step we observe, evaluate, and label. It's an efficient way of organizing the world as we grow up. We eat an orange. We feel nourished and delighted. We judge the orange tasty. And we declare it a good orange.

"Observing without evaluating is the highest form of human intelligence."

J. Krishnamurti

But that same skill often gets in the way as we interact with other people. We see socks on the floor. We're uncomfortable because we want order. We judge the person who left them there as sloppy and label him a bad roommate.

Your patients are observing your behavior, evaluating it, and labeling you all the time. A patient feels a needle miss the vein. He feels pain and uncertainty. He judges the nurse as careless and labels her inept.

You and your fellow staff members are the subject of a lot of judgments. Each time you sense or hear a judgment, your choice of how to respond helps shape the eventual outcome of your interaction.

Here's another opportunity to put yourself in your patient's place. Imagine you have the experience below and you make a judgment as a result. Listen for how the caregiver responds to you, and think where it will likely lead the interaction.

41

You are 50 years old and an avid runner. You've had a persistent sore throat for the past few weeks and you've been short of breath for the past two. Last week your doctor felt "a small obstruction" in your throat and referred you to a specialist. Following a biopsy, your specialist told you that you had cancer with an indeterminate prognosis and checked you into a cancer service at a nearby hospital.

A surgeon and a respiratory therapist (RT) arrive at your room together. The doctor looks over a CT scan and biopsy, feels your throat, announces that he'll schedule a laryngectomy later the same morning, and leaves.

After you talk through your shock, you remark about the physician, "Wow, he is so arrogant."

As you read the therapist's responses, write down your gut reaction in the spaces below. (There is no right or wrong reaction. Your reaction is true for you.) Once again, you'll find the strategies in [brackets] to make them easy to identify:

RT: He's really not such a bad guy. And he's a brilliant surgeon [defending].

How you feel inside as the patient hearing this response:

_____

_____

_____

_____

RT: He only did that because he has such a tight schedule [explaining].

How you feel inside as the patient hearing this response:

_____

_____

_____

_____

RT: I'm sorry, that really was arrogant wasn't it? [commiserating].

How you feel inside as the patient hearing this response:

_____

_____

_____

_____

Again, you'll have your own reactions. When we've used this scenario in the past, people tend to see the first two responses as dismissive. And it's common for the interaction to escalate into a confrontation.

Commiserating can create some short-term connection between the RT and the patient but it doesn't help the RT figure out how to foster a better experience for the patient. And painting the patient as a victim can increase the risk for your organization.

See how much more helpful the RT can be simply by clarifying the observation that's driving the patient in the first place.

Patient: "Wow, he is so arrogant."

RT: "Are you reacting to him scheduling an operation without checking with you?"

Patient: "No, I trust his judgment. If I need the operation, I want it. But you'd think he'd spend a minute with me if he's going to have his hands in my throat."

The RT still has some important things to work out. But instead of having a patient who's learning to think of herself as a victim, the RT has a patient with a need he can propose solutions for.

Ways to help your patients clarify their observations

1. Clarify the actions they've observed that are at the source of their judgments
2. Clarify the specific time and context of observations that they are expressing as generalizations

ALIVE doesn't require that your patients stop judging. It does suggest that you both will have better interactions and outcomes when you help patients separate their observations from their evaluations.

In the examples that follow, note how the caregiver's questions help identify the source of the patients' judgments so you can work toward effective action.

Example #1

Patient: I'm a terrible wife. I'm such a burden.

Caregiver: Is this about hearing that you need an operation?

Example #2

Patient: That other nurse is so disorganized.

Caregiver: Are you reacting to her saying she doesn't know who was on shift last night?

Example #3

Patient: You've got to do something about that girl in the next bed. She's impossible!

Caregiver: Is it the number of visitors your roommate had in here this afternoon that concerns you?

Example #4

Patient: You're never on time!

Caregiver: Are you responding to my being 10 minutes late for our last two appointments?

When you ask about observations, you're trying to identify what your patient has seen, heard, or reflected on that has affected their experience of life.

You'll put the question in your own words.

∴ "Are you responding to…"

∴ "Are you thinking of…"

∴ "Are you reacting to…"

∴ "Is this about…"

Your goal is to identify the observation behind the judgment. Clarifying what your patient has observed will put you in a better position to take action. And separating the observation from your patient's interpretation will make it less likely that you'll hear yourself being judged.

For the following examples, try writing responses that help your patient identify what they've seen or heard that leads to their evaluations:

1. An operation like that is a waste on a guy like me.

_____

2. I'm just one more bed to you folks, aren't I?

_____

3. He thinks he's such a big shot.

_____

4. I'm getting worse. I'm not getting any better.

_____

Here are some answers we liked.

1. An operation like that is a waste on a guy like me.
   Is it something you heard about your possible outcomes that leaves you concerned?

2. I'm just one more bed to you folks, aren't I?
   Are you thinking about your upcoming discharge?

3. He thinks he's such a big shot.
   Are you reacting to him walking out after three minutes?

4. I'm getting worse. I'm not getting any better.
   Is it the six pounds you've lost?

These are very likely not the answers you've given. And they may or may not be what the patient meant. It's not important that you guess correctly about what your patient is thinking, but that you demonstrate your interest in him. And you do it in a way that underscores that his experience arises from his observations.

In responding to question 2, for example, an answer such as "So, you're concerned that you're just a number to us" is essentially parroting the original statement, while a statement such as one we've provided attempts to identify what the patient has seen or heard that gives rise to their reaction.

Make it real

What judgments or generalizations do you hear often?
Think of three judgments or generalizations you hear regularly from your patients. Write down a question you might ask to help them clarify *the actions they've observed* that are at the source of their judgments or *the specific time and*

context of observations that they are expressing as generalizations.

For example, Roger often hears complaints about the scheduling. "You folks are always running so far behind!" He could ask, "Are you anxious at hearing it will be 5 weeks before your next visit?"

1. Judgment or generalization you often hear:

_____

_____

"Analyses of other human beings are tragic expressions of our own values and needs."

Question you could ask to clarify the observation:

_____

_____

Marshall Rosenberg

2. Judgment or generalization you often hear:

_____

_____

_____

Question you could ask to clarify the observation:

_____

_____

_____

3. Judgment or generalization you often hear:

_____

_____

_____

Question you could ask to clarify the observation:

_____

_____

_____

Attending to Emotions

Listening for your patient's FEELINGS

The first step in the process of verifying what's alive is helping your patient clarify what he's observing that's affecting his well-being. As part of that step, you'll want to help him separate those observations from his judgments about them. The second step is to help your patient clarify the feelings he's having that are triggered by what he's observing.

We often overlook the power of simply acknowledging the feelings of another. Our feelings are an indication of what we're going through and of how intense our experience is. Sometimes, just speaking your patients' feelings out loud is enough to open up a deeper level of connection.

Asking, "You're really feeling low, aren't you?" or saying, "I hear how frustrated you are, even angry…" can be all you need to do to let your patients know that your paying attention to them, that you're interested in how they are.

"Sometimes, just speaking your patients' feelings out loud is enough to open up a deeper level of connection."

An experience I had training some respiratory therapists demonstrates how reluctant we can be to admit feelings into our conversations.

The head of the group brought in a scenario for us to work through. It involved a 28-year-old woman recovering from a gall stone operation. As a start, I asked one of the therapists we were training to enter the patient's room and acknowledge the patient's feelings whatever they were.

When the therapist entered her room, the patient told him her name, spelled her last name, and reminded him of her room number. The therapist checked and noted all the information.

51

As he began his assessment, the patient interrupted him to ask him to pour her some water, unpack some food she'd received from her brother, rub her feet, and shift her pillows. He did all these things as the other therapists who were observing visibly squirmed. The patient went so far as to ask the therapist to go down to the admin office to settle a billing problem she was having. He finally balked at this request and excused himself.

When I asked the group how the woman seemed, they erupted with pent up opinions. She's upset, uncomfortable, cross, stern, edgy. The group had a variety of suggestions for handling the encounter differently. One therapist stepped up and exclaimed, "You really have to set boundaries with a person like that!"

Not one of them suggested that we acknowledge what the patient was feeling.

"Most of us have a limited vocabulary for expressing how we feel. Yet, we have a large repertoire of words that communicate what we think and how we think others are treating us."

Earlier in the day, the patient had received a blood draw scheduled for a patient in another room down the hall. We were talking about setting boundaries for her. And all the while, she was trying to establish some boundaries and control of her own.

All it took to open up that conversation was a straightforward question: "You seem a little uncomfortable to me, are you apprehensive about something?" But the therapists seemed to feel a prohibition against mentioning feelings even after I had invited them to.

Even when we address feelings openly, our language creates confusion and fosters confrontation. Most of us have a limited vocabulary for expressing how we feel. Yet, we have a large repertoire of words that communicate what we think and how we think others are treating us.

For example, whenever we run a training program, we

include a scenario in which a caregiver laments that she's not cut out for the job and should quit. When I ask the group how the caregiver is feeling, I get a range of answers: she feels like she's a failure, or she feels as if she can't do the job. She feels *inadequate* or *unimportant*.

Though these are all someone's interpretations of what the caregiver is going though, none of them is an expression of feeling. When words such as *like, that,* and *as if* follow the word *feel* the thing being expressed is a thought, not a feeling. Words like *inadequate* or *unimportant* aren't feelings. They're judgments we make of ourselves.

I'll also hear that she feels *isolated, abandoned, neglected, overworked,* and *taken for granted*. We often take these as feelings, but none of them is. They're expressions of how we think other people are treating us—isolating me, abandoning me, neglecting me, etc.

To identify patients' feelings, you really don't need a lot of rules. In fact, we just ask for a gut reaction. That usually produces a feeling word—sad, mad, glad, or afraid.

This is a problem with manuals that advise you to "validate your patient's feelings." You can end up validating your patient's judgments and their picture of themselves as victims instead. Patients will see themselves as less empowered and less at the center of their own care. You'll wonder why you don't feel the warmth of having contributed. And your organization will be at greater risk.

The way we separate true feelings from our confusing language about feelings is to ask simply, "And when you think that, how do you feel?" For example, you say you feel *as if you deserve better*. I ask,

∴ When you think that, how do you feel?

Cheated.

∴ When you think that, how do you feel?

Despondent.

∴ When you think that, how do you feel?

Just *despondent*.

Then you're at a base feeling.

Here's a list of words and phrases that we substitute for feelings that aren't really feelings.

Thoughts disguised as feelings.

I feel:

∴ that, like, as if (these are explaining words that introduce thoughts)

∴ I, you, he, she, they, it, Jerry, my patient, my boss (these are pronouns that introduce judgments**)**

Judgments about ourselves disguised as feelings.

I feel:

∴ Inadequate, incompetent, inappropriate, unacceptable

Descriptions of how we think others are treating us disguised as feelings

I feel:

∴ Unimportant, disrespected, misunderstood and the whole list of verbs that end in 'ed' or begin in 'un' such as −

abandoned	distrusted	put down
abused	interrupted	rejected
attacked	intimidated	taken for granted
betrayed	let down	threatened

"When people are trying not to feel an emotion, they perceive themselves practically to be victims of the feeling and of whomever or whatever is stimulating it."

Jim Leonard

bullied	manipulated	unappreciated
cheated	neglected	unheard
coerced	overworked	unsupported
cornered	patronized	unwanted
diminished	pressured	used

Authentic feelings

The authentic feelings revolve around just four emotions—
glad, mad, sad, and afraid—and the physical sensations in
the body. Generally, we'll feel some variation on glad and
physically vigorous when we're getting our needs met.

absorbed	courageous	friendly	keyed-up	safe
adventurous	curious	fulfilled	lively	satisfied
affectionate	delighted	glad	loving	secure
alert	eager	gleeful	mellow	sensitive
alive	ebullient	glorious	merry	serene
amused	ecstatic	glowing	mirthful	spellbound
appreciative	effervescent	good-humored	moved	splendid
aroused	elated	grateful	optimistic	stimulated
astonished	enchanted	hopeful	overjoyed	surprised
blissful	energetic	inquisitive	peaceful	tender
buoyant	engrossed	inspired	perky	thankful
calm	enthusiastic	intense	pleasant	thrilled
carefree	excited	interested	pleased	touched
cheerful	exhilarated	intrigued	radiant	tranquil
comfortable	expectant	invigorated	rapturous	upbeat

composed	exultant	involved	refreshed	warm
confident	fascinated	joyous, joyful	relaxed	wide awake
contented	free	jubilant	relieved	wonderful

And we'll feel some variety of sad, mad, or afraid and
physically depleted when our needs are going unmet.

afraid	despondent	fidgety	lethargic	skeptical
aggravated	detached	gloomy	listless	sleepy
agitated	disaffected	guilty	mopey	sorrowful
alarmed	disenchanted	harried	morose	suspicious
aloof	disappointed	heavy	mournful	tepid
angry	discouraged	helpless	nervous	terrified
anguished	disgruntled	hesitant	nettled	tired
annoyed	disgusted	horrified	numb	troubled
anxious	disheartened	horrible	overwhelmed	uncomfortable
apathetic	dismayed	hostile	panicky	uncertain
apprehensive	displeased	hot	passive	uneasy
ashamed	disquieted	humdrum	perplexed	unglued
beat	distressed	hurt	pessimistic	unhappy
bewildered	disturbed	impatient	puzzled	unnerved
bitter	downcast	indifferent	rancorous	unsteady
blah	downhearted	intense	reluctant	upset
blue	dull	irate	repelled	uptight
bored	edgy	irked	resentful	vexed
brokenhearted	embarrassed	irritated	restless	weary
chagrined	embittered	jealous	sad	wistful

cold	exasperated	jittery	scared	withdrawn
concerned	exhausted	keyed-up	shaky	woeful
confused	fatigued	leery	shocked	worried
depressed	frightened	mad	spiritless	wretched

In the examples below, the caregiver guesses how her patient is feeling.

Example #1

Patient: Well, I'm not sure about another operation. I was really for it when you brought it up before. But now, you know…

Caregiver: Are you feeling uncertain about what to do next?

Example #2

Patient: Yeah, I'm taking all the drugs. But I don't know that they're doing anything.

Caregiver: You sound as though you may be a little anxious.

Example #3

Patient: I feel like she isn't listening to me. I feel really ignored.

Caregiver: I hear your frustration and I wonder if you're a bit worried too.

Notice these are only guesses. You don't have to become a mind reader to use the ALIVE model. The purpose of this step is to demonstrate your intention to connect with your patient and help your patient clarify his feelings. That's often a process of trial and error.

Put it into action

Below you'll see a series of statements that patients might make. For each one, write a word or two that indicates how your patient might be feeling (again, you'll need to guess). Then, write a statement that demonstrates to your patient that your intention is to understand his feelings.

For example, a patient might say, "Can't you just use plain English instead of all that mumbo-jumbo?" A word that describes how he might be feeling is *confused*. You might demonstrate your attention to his feelings by saying, "The technical descriptions can be kind of confusing, can't they?"

1. **I don't know what good it does for you to give me these prescriptions when I can't even afford them.**

   Word that describes how your patient might be feeling

   _____

   A statement that demonstrates you are attending to your

   patient's feelings_____

   _____

   _____

2. **I have 17 days clean. So, that's good, right?**

   Word that describes how your patient might be feeling

   _____

   A statement that demonstrates you are attending to your

   patient's feelings_____

   _____

   _____

3. **So, what you're telling me is that you aren't going to admit me, despite the pain.**

   Word that describes how your patient might be feeling

   _____

   A statement that demonstrates you are attending to your

   patient's feelings_____

   _____

4. **My white count has really been solid these past couple of months. I hold on to that.**

   Word that describes how your patient might be feeling

   _____

   A statement that demonstrates you are attending to your

   patient's feelings_____

   _____

   _____

Here are some answers we liked.

1. *I don't know what good it does for you to give me these prescriptions when I can't even afford them.*

    ∴ Word that describes how your patient might be feeling:
    worried

    ∴ A statement that demonstrates you are attending to your patient's feelings:
    Are you a little worried about how you're going to pay for these?

2. *I have 17 days clean. So, that's good, right?*

    ∴ Word that describes how your patient might be feeling:
    proud

    ∴ A statement that demonstrates you are attending to your patient's feelings:
    I see you're proud of what you've been able to do.

3. *So, what you're telling me is that you aren't going to admit me, despite the pain.*

    ∴ Word that describes how your patient might be feeling:
    uneasy

    ∴ A statement that demonstrates you are attending to your patient's feelings:
    You're uneasy about going home?

4. *My white count has really been solid these past couple of months. I hold onto that.*

    ∴ Word that describes how your patient might be feeling:
    hopeful

∴ A statement that demonstrates you are attending to your patient's feelings:

So, you're feeling pretty hopeful about that.

Getting to the Core

Identifying the NEEDS at the root of your patients' experience

We've been working a lot with judgments and criticisms, what your patients may be saying about you or about themselves. The most powerful insight for you—if you're going to foster better experiences for yourself and your patients—is that all statements like these are tragic expressions of needs.

"Understanding human needs is half the job of meeting them."

Adlai Stevenson, Jr.

∴ If a patient says, "You people are so slow, this is the worst I've ever seen," she's telling you she needs consideration for her time.

∴ When a family member says, "He's just another patient to you, but he's all I've got," he's telling you he needs to be able to trust that his father is getting the attention he needs.

∴ When a patient says, "You're a racist," she's saying she has a need for fairness or to be treated as an individual.

And those needs are currently going unmet.

Unfortunately, just as most of us use "feeling" words to express our thoughts, "I feel like you folks are always running late," we also use "need" words to express demands, "You need to make my appointment right now!"

Our habitual patterns of language lead us to believe we have to strong-arm other people to get our needs met.

The underlying logic goes like this: if I'm not getting my needs met, you must be wrong, and you need to change. For example, If I need more peace and rest in the room, I call you inconsiderate for having all those visitors in. If I need more confidence that I'm getting good medical attention, I tell you you're uncaring or unprofessional.

Why we feel what we feel

Read over the following dialogue paying attention to the mother's feelings. List those feelings on the left-hand side of the table below. On the right hand, write down what caused her to feel that way.

A medical unit is working with a black family. They think the patient's impending discharge will be welcome news to the family. Instead, the boy's mother reacts with anger. "You aren't hearing me, but you're gonna. You're taking care of my son until he gets better. Why are you tryin' to hustle us outta here? Why do you people treat me this way? You come in here in pairs and you won't look me in the eye. Do I even have to say it? You wouldn't be treating me this way if I were white. Why don't you just get outta my room?"

The mother feels	Because
1.	
2.	
3.	

On the following page, you'll see the kind of list many people would create.

Here's a list typical of what we see in training.

The mother feels	Because
1. Angry	The hospital staff come in pairs and won't look in her eyes.
2. Unhappy	She doesn't get any respect
3. Upset	The staff hasn't adequately prepped her for her son's discharge.

The key misunderstanding

The kinds of reasons you see listed above in the right-hand column will tend to get in the way of creating a good experience with the mother. Our language misleads us into thinking that other people are responsible for our emotions and our experience of life. How often have you heard, "You make me so mad when you…"

"Our language misleads us into thinking that other people are responsible for our emotions and our experience of life".

The mother was angry WHEN the staff came into her room in pairs—but not BECAUSE the staff came into her room in pairs.

Staff members have surely entered other rooms in pairs. Each of those patients reacted differently depending on their needs and expectations. Some who wanted extra attention may have been delighted. Others who saw it as a defensive move on the part of the caregivers may have felt guilty. This mother reacted with anger.

If the staff members didn't make the mother angry, neither did the mother make the staff defensive. **No one makes another person feel any way**. Your actions may be a stimulus for the feelings of others.

But ultimately, **our feelings are a product of our own needs and expectations**.

So, how can you help your patients break out of this cycle?

There are two things you can do:

1. Listen for a call for help. ALIVE reminds you that your patients' feelings and their criticisms arise from their own needs and expectations. Focus your attention on their needs, and you'll be less likely to get defensive yourself.

2. Translate your patients' evaluations and judgments in a way that reveals the connection between their feelings and their underlying needs and expectations.

Listen for a call for help

When someone, say the mother in the previous example, makes a negative statement, you can *choose* how you hear it.

You can play "The Blame Game" or become a "Needs Detective."

The mother says, "You're not listening to me but you're gonna!" Let's look at how your choice of ways to listen determines your response.

The Blame Game

You can choose to take the comment personally and attack or defend.

If you blame yourself, you'll accept the criticism and apologize, "I'm sorry, I didn't mean to disturb you. Maybe I can come back later."

If you blame your patient, you'll find fault with her. That might lead you to say, for example, "I assure you that you're son's care is my highest concern" while thinking to yourself, "Right now, your attitude and behavior are interfering with that care."

When you accept the criticism, you'll feel guilt or shame. When you blame your patient, you'll become angry. All those emotions are likely to come between you and the quality of experience you want to create.

Four Ways You Can Choose to Hear Negative Comments	
Blame yourself and take on guilt	Blame the other person and build up resentment
Focus on your own needs and reveal your humanity	Focus on the other person's needs and demonstrate empathy

The Needs Detective

Alternatively, you can tune into the needs that are going unmet.

When you turn your attention to your own needs, you can reveal your humanity, "When I hear you talk that way, I'm frustrated that I'm working hard and not getting the results I'd hoped for."

When you turn your attention to your patient's needs, you can demonstrate your empathy, "Are you anxious about getting the support you need?"

You might think it would be tough for your patients to listen to your needs and feelings. And I'd agree with you much of the time. If she's giving you judgments and accusations, your patient likely has important needs to satisfy before she'll be a good audience for you.

Surprisingly, though, many patients are aching to hear what's alive in you, especially if it's a reaction to them. It reminds them you're human and lets them know they're having an effect on you. We'll talk about that more in Section Three: Taking a Stand.

Again, you don't have to become a mind reader to use ALIVE. The purpose of this step is metaphorically move over to the patient's side of the table, to demonstrate your intention to connect with your patient, and help your patient identify his needs. That's often a process of trial and error.

Getting the first guess right isn't your goal. Showing a sincere interest is.

Translating your patients' judgments to reveal the connection between feelings and needs

We want patients to be as empowered as possible in their healing process. Our habitual language works against that empowerment by making it appear that you are the cause of their feelings.

You can help your patients by clarifying the connection between their feelings and their needs. See which of these two responses leave your patient seeing herself as most empowered.

Caregiver: So, I made you mad by showing up late with your medication?

OR…

Caregiver: So, you were mad when I showed up at 8:25 with your medication because you were hoping for some quiet time with your husband.

Few options arise out of the first response. Essentially, your patient can't be happy until you become more punctual.

The second response puts your patient at the center of her own experience. You trace her anger to her own unfulfilled desire for connection with her husband.

This is also a more accurate description. Imagine how grateful she might be to you if you had interrupted a conversation that was unpleasant for her or if she'd been hoping to introduce her husband to you. It also leads naturally to a discussion of options for getting your patient what she needs.

Needs: the heart of your relationship with patients

Needs are the core of this whole process. But what do we mean by needs, anyway? Needs are the basic human necessities. And you'll foster better experiences by avoiding a common misunderstanding: the confusion of needs with strategies.

It may be helpful to think of needs as falling into four categories.

To live safely and survive	To love and be loved	To be true to yourself	To thrive and see possibility
safety	community	autonomy	unity
security	connection	authenticity	purpose
food	cooperation	creativity	fun, play, joy
water	empathy	freedom, choice	possibility
shelter	consideration	learning	meaning
health	reassurance	honesty	celebration
rest	to be seen	challenge	inspiration
ease	to be heard	self-expression	contribution
harmony	acceptance	space	beauty
peace	trust	clarity	mourning

The critical Difference

Needs are:	Strategies are:
Universal human drives, motivations, and longings	*Specific* solutions tied to a person taking an action
Examples: ∴ Autonomy (to have choice) ∴ Cooperation ∴ Peace	Examples: ∴ Let me see my doctor now ∴ Give me a private room ∴ Come back in twenty minutes

Impasses arise from a clash of competing strategies.

You don't have that problem with needs. Each party can advocate for his or her own needs and expect support from the other (as long as they have trust and rapport).

Compare the dialogues that follow. The first is a disagreement over strategies. The second is a discussion of needs.

Example #1

Caregiver: "You have to be quiet in this zone"

Patient: "It's part of my culture to raise my voice when I'm angry. I have a right to speak my mind, and I'm going to stay here till I do."

Example #2

Caregiver: "It's important to me to provide a space with harmony where our patients can recuperate."

Patient: "It's critical to me to speak my side of the story and be heard out."

The more forcefully we argue for a strategy the more stubborn we seem. The more forcefully we present our needs, the more we reveal intensity of our concerns.

Here are some examples of caregivers translating patient's comments into a language of needs. In these statements, the caregivers identify their patients' needs and the connection between those needs and their patients' feelings.

Example #1

Patient: I get really upset when you make mistakes like that. You just can't do that.

Caregiver: It's important to you to know that you're getting a high quality of care.

Example #2

Patient: I deserve better treatment than this. This is the most inconvenient place to come!

Caregiver: You're irritated because your time really matters to you and you'd like your visits to be easier?

Example #3

Patient: You may work here, but you don't know anything about me or my people.

Caregiver: This is upsetting for you. You want to be recognized for who you are.

Example #4

Patient: I feel totally neglected and taken for granted.

Caregiver: You're very frustrated because you want to be valued and to get the attention you need.

The gift in victim language

Remember, in the previous unit we talked about "descriptions of how we think others are treating us" that go disguised as feelings. We included phrases such as I feel *abandoned*, *cheated*, *pressured*, or *unappreciated*. We made the point in that unit that these words aren't feelings at all. Now we can name them as **expressions of unmet needs**.

When you hear expressions like these, all you need to do to identify the unmet need is to think of the opposite of how they say they feel. Here are some examples:

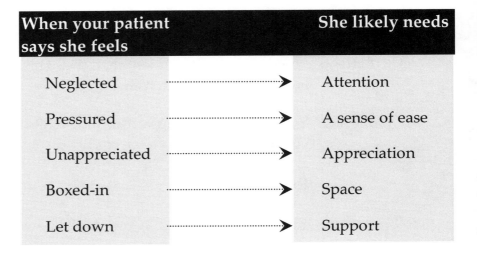

When your patient says she feels		She likely needs
Neglected	⟶	Attention
Pressured	⟶	A sense of ease
Unappreciated	⟶	Appreciation
Boxed-in	⟶	Space
Let down	⟶	Support

You Try

Below you'll see a series of statements that patients might make. For each one, write out how you'd respond if you were choosing to focus on your patient's needs rather than getting caught up in blame.

1. **You really irritate me, keeping me waiting like this.**

   How you'd respond if you chose to focus on your patient's needs

   _____

   _____

2. **I feel like you're abandoning me, you know, saying I should stop treatment.**

   How you'd respond if you chose to focus on your patient's needs

   _____

   _____

3. **What is this? This shouldn't be on my bill.**

   How you'd respond if you chose to focus on your patient's needs

   _____

   _____

4. **Oh, you're gonna tell me how I feel now, huh? OK, how do I feel?**

   How you'd respond if you chose to focus on your patient's needs

   _____

   _____

Here are some answers we liked:

1. You really irritate me, keeping me waiting like this.

   ∴ How you'd respond if you chose to focus on your patient's needs

   You'd like some recognition for how important your time is.

2. I feel like you're abandoning me, you know, saying I should stop treatment.

   ∴ How you'd respond if you chose to focus on your patient's needs

   I can hear your despair. You need to know that you're not alone, that you'll still get support and attention through this experience.

3. What is this? This shouldn't be on my bill.

   ∴ How you'd respond if you chose to focus on your patient's needs

   You're frustrated because you want to be treated fairly and understand why we're charging what we are.

4. Oh, you're gonna tell me how I feel now, huh? OK, how do I feel?

   ∴ How you'd respond if you chose to focus on your patient's needs

   You really want to be seen and heard for who you are.

Again, you may not phrase your responses this way. In fact, these responses may not be what the patient is looking for. What's important is to demonstrate that you're focusing on him, and to underscore that it's his own needs that give rise to his feelings.

Feelings! Oh, my life of feelings!

Feelings are an indicator of internal experience. They tell you whether your patient is getting his needs met and how intense his experience is.

When he's getting his needs met a little, he's likely comfortable. When he's getting his needs met thoroughly, he's exuberant.

When he's not getting his needs met, he may be irritated or annoyed. When he has deep needs that are completely unmet, he's furious or despondent.

Identifying feelings can help you anticipate your patients' needs and create rapport. But for most patients, it's just a first step. People who've just told you how they feel often don't need to have it reflected back to them.

Patient: "I'm angry!"

Caregiver: "So, you're saying you're pretty mad."

If you look at the exercises above, you'll see that we generally call out feelings when patients don't reveal them. Once your patients know you understand whether they're getting their needs met and to what degree, they'll want to move on to talking about those needs.

Would you like me to...

Encouraging REQUESTS that enrich life

The first three units of this Section cover the heart of the ALIVE model—Verify what's alive. We've recommended up to this point that you consciously avoid talk of what we've called strategies—specific solutions that involve particular people. There are two reasons.

First, starting with strategies invites conflict. Focusing on feelings and needs will put you on common ground with your patients; it will reveal your common humanity. Second, you'll be better able to come up with strategies that work for everyone once you've clarified the needs.

We began by separating your patients' observations from their judgments. Then we called out their feelings. We've also learned how to translate habitual language to uncover your patients' needs. Using these skills will help you avoid hearing criticism and blame.

In this unit, we'll discuss the final step of the ALIVE model, **E**ncourage a request that enriches life. We'll lay out a few simple reminders you can use to help your patients form requests that work for them, for you, and for your organization.

We'll look at three things you can do that will help you fashion requests with your patients most effectively:

1. Verify your patients' needs before you help them form requests

2. Make implied requests explicit, and

3. Form specific requests for action.

"Patients reserve their good word of mouth and loyalty for hospitals where they feel their needs were anticipated and met by a courteous, caring staff."

Fred Lee

Verify your patients' needs before you help them form requests

Caregivers are wonderful problem solvers. And with the wealth of experience you bring to work everyday, you can probably spot problems and corresponding solutions very quickly. Ironically, this can stand between you and a good relationship with some patients. Here's an example.

I was coaching a nurse through an interaction with a father who was outraged. He thought the staff was trying to hustle him and his son out of the hospital. I pulled the nurse aside just after the man blew up at her. He had told her that he worked all day and came into the hospital all night. And where did she think he was going to get the time to go through training before he took his son home?

"First, he needed to know that he was seen as an individual with unique concerns."

When I asked her how she thought the man was feeling and what he needed, she suggested to me that he seemed overwhelmed and afraid, and that he might need some support. When I suggested she ask the man if that's what he was experiencing, she turned to him and said, "You need an appointment with a social worker. I'll set something up for you."

Not surprisingly, he blew up again.

He actually needed a social worker. In fact, when we finished talking with him, the solution we settled on was just that.

The father pushed back because he wasn't ready to hear a solution even though the nurse was ready to suggest it. The father needed a social worker, yes. But first, he needed to know that he was seen as an individual with unique concerns.

We don't see this in every case, but it's often true in those encounters where your habitual responses don't work for you. The patient or family member needs more trust, or acknowledgement of the difficult time they've had. And they need it before they can move on to solutions.

There are two ways to resolve a situation like this. The first is to take the process at the patient's speed. Check out your observations and opinions with your patient before you propose solutions.

Caregiver: "This seems a little overwhelming, doesn't it? You look like you might welcome some support. Would you like me to see about setting up an appointment with a social worker so you can find some support that works for you?"

The second way to handle this kind of situation is to propose the solution you think makes sense and give empathy if your patient isn't ready.

Caregiver: "You need an appointment with a social worker. I'll set something up for you."

Patient: "You aren't hearing me. We're not going anywhere!"

Caregiver: "Are you angry because you need some time to work this through and some recognition for how challenging this is?"

You give empathy until you have rapport again. And then you help your patient form a request that meets their needs.

Make implied requests explicit

The core of this process is recognizing that each of us is trying to get our needs met all the time. We're making requests of each other whether those requests are implied in our behavior or explicitly stated out loud.

Remember the woman in Unit 2 of this Section. She repeated the room number when her RT came in, repeated her name, and spelled it. We can **hear those actions as requests**—"Tell me you know who I am. Tell me I can rest assured you're here for me."

We can even hear a broader context for the requests she spoke. When she said, "Arrange my pillow, bring me water, and massage my feet," she might also have been saying, "let me know I still have some say in what happens to my body."

The solution, as in the example above, is to give empathy until you understand the patient's needs, and then help them form a request to meet those needs.

Form specific requests for action

As you help patients form requests, it's important that you become clear about what they want so you both will recognize when they've received it. Take these patient requests as an example.

"You all need to show me more respect."

"Stop being late all the time!"

"I've got to be more involved in the decisions around my treatment plan."

All of these are worthwhile sentiments. None of them is a well-formed request. They're wishes. And wishes won't help. Because even if you agree, you may not know how to deliver. Even "stop being late" is too

Requests that are too general	Requests specific enough to work
"You'd like me to stop hedging about your condition."	"You'd like me to show you your test results and answer your questions until you say you understand."
"You'd like to be treated with more respect."	"You'd like us to look you in the eyes, and call you by name."
"You'd like some recognition for your convictions as a Muslim."	"You'd like a meeting with food service where you can see the diet and sign off on your plan."

general. We want to be clear about **the behavior a patient will see** that will satisfy them they are getting what they need.

The solution is simple. Ask your patient how she'll know when she's gotten what she wants. And don't settle until you have specific answers.

Here are some examples of caregivers translating patients' comments into specific requests. In these statements, the caregivers identify their patients' needs and the connection between those needs and their patients' feelings.

Example #1

Patient: Would you please show me some respect for my privacy.

Caregiver: Would you rather meet in my office to finish discussing your medical options at this point?

Example #2

Patient: You've got to consider my family's schedule sometimes.

Caregiver: Would you like to talk to the charge nurse about scheduling some exceptions to the policies on visitation?

Example #3

Patient: I'm an old man you know. It would be nice if you'd take that into account.

Caregiver: Would it be helpful if we sent someone to the curb to help you out of your car?

Example #4

Patient: So you're saying I've got to stop smoking.

Caregiver: I'd like to chat with you about what you get out of smoking and how you can get those needs met in ways that are healthier for you.

Pin it down!

Below you'll see a series of statements that patients might make. For each one, write out how you'd make the request clear enough that you both would recognize **the action you'd need to take** to satisfy their needs.

1. **I'll tell you what would help, a consistent story. You tell me this; she tells me that; he tells me another thing.**

   How you'd clarify the request so you recognize the actions you need to take

   _____

2. **I'd like to know you're taking my needs into account.**

   How you'd clarify the request so you recognize the actions you need to take

   _____

3. **You've got to keep me in the loop on these decisions. You just can't keep going around me.**

   How you'd clarify the request so you recognize the actions you need to take

   _____

4. **Well, you could start by charging reasonable amounts for these services.**

   How you'd clarify the request so you recognize the actions you need to take

   _____

Here are some answers we liked:

1. I'll tell you what would help, a consistent story. You tell me this; she tells me that; he tells me another thing.

   ∴ How you'd clarify the request so you recognize the actions you need to take

   Would you like to schedule a time the four of us can sit down together to talk this though?

2. I'd like to know you're taking my needs into account.

   ∴ How you'd clarify the request so you recognize the actions you need to take

   Would you like me to tell you what I heard you say?

3. You've got to keep me in the loop on these decisions. You just can't keep going around me.

   ∴ How you'd clarify the request so you recognize the actions you need to take

   Would you like to work with me to set up a process so that you sign off when we suggest changes in treatment?

4. Well, you could start by charging reasonable amounts for these services.

   ∴ How you'd clarify the request so you recognize the actions you need to take

   Would you like to schedule a time to meet with bookkeeping so you can review the charges on your bill?

Bringing it ALIVE

OK, you've seen the model end-to-end. Now, how do you put it to use on the job?

That depends on you and your personality. You're already adept at working with patients.

Often these empathy skills will show up just as they have in the exercises—as a simple comment, something you say in passing when you want to deepen rapport with a patient. You'll be making a visible statement of your intention to focus on your patient.

"Often these empathy skills will show up simply as a comment, something you say in passing when you want to deepen rapport with a patient."

Sometimes, you'll notice that the responses that normally work with patients aren't working for you. You'll notice your rapport deteriorating even as you're trying to help. In those cases, ALIVE can help you negotiate that 'dance' you enter into with patients, the give and take of building a relationship.

You'll find below, an example of how that worked for a unit we trained.

A teen-aged boy was recovering from a stay in a critical care unit. His parents had requested that no information be given out about their son and that he receive no visitors. The parents fought, occasionally loudly, and were put off at working with new nurses.

Here's a typical interaction with Bill, the father, before the staff learned the skills.

Bill: I left the room for a few minutes and you let in that stir-fry. My son's a vegetarian. You just picked the chicken out. The vegetables are already contaminated. What part of vegetarian don't you understand?

Nurse: I'm sorry the food wasn't right. You sound very concerned. I can set up an appointment for you with dietary so that doesn't happen again.

Bill: Well-good. But what about the noise in here? Listen to that! This is the loudest place I've ever been.

Nurse: It is loud isn't it? I can see if you can get a private room. Would you like that?

Bill: It would be nice. It's bad enough with new nurses coming through here at all hours.

Nurse: I see why you'd be upset. You really need some consistency don't you.

Bill: Well, of course I do. Did you see that troupe of kids that came in this morning? That's no good. How did they get in here? I've got to have some control over who comes into this room.

It won't surprise you that the staff was frightened to work with the family. Confrontations were common and they often escalated.

You'll notice this isn't your common encounter. The nurse is continually offering solutions. Yet, Bill holds onto to his anger and frustration. That's a good sign that he could benefit from some active empathy. ALIVE is a good fit for this interaction.

Assess your rapport

Listen for a call for help

Intend to connect

Verify what's alive

Encourage a request that enriches life

Here's an example of how we coached the nurse to use the skills with this family. You'll notice that the nurse doesn't use pat phrases. She weaves the model into her own style of talking which includes her own observations. Also, notice that we don't move straight through the model. We're constantly revisiting steps to refocus our attention and see if we're creating the experience we want.

Bill: Did you see that troupe of kids that came in this morning? That's no good. How did they get in here? I've got to have some control over who comes into this room.

Nurse: You sound very agitated. We can set things up so that you're informed about any changes and you have sign off for as much of this as possible.

Bill: (under his breath) Yeah, it's about time.

Coach: OK, let's pause briefly. You're validating Bill's requests and offering solutions. And yet he still seems angry. I'd say that's a sign that you don't have the rapport with him that you're hoping for. Would you agree?

Nurse: If you're asking if I'm feeling good about this, then no, I'm not.

Coach: Ok, you're solving his son's problems. What might Bill need? Why don't you try focusing on him a moment?

Nurse: Bill, you look just exhausted to me. Are you feeling really tired?

Bill: Oh God, yes. You've seen me. I'm in here everyday. I sleep right here on this chair every night.

Nurse: I want to tell him that I can find a place for him to sleep but my suggestions haven't seemed to make him very happy so far.

Coach: Yeah, I'd agree with your intuition. You might check your understanding of his need—rest, a break, some relief—before you move on to a specific solution. It's a small difference. But he might feel more heard.

Nurse: (to Bill) You look like you could use some kind of relief.

Bill: Yeah, I do. (Bill's face visibly relaxes.) But how can I? (His face and posture tighten up again.) I leave for a few minutes and my son gets food he can't eat. He's just a patient to you, but he's my boy, you know. The only one I have. And you know my wife hardly ever makes it in. So there's no one else. I've got to be here to watch you people.

Nurse: OK, that hurt. I want to tell him that it wasn't my fault, that he can trust us. But I don't think he'll believe it.

Coach: I agree. He may not be ready to hear that. Why don't you stay focused on his needs? Notice how that helped you create connection. He can acknowledge a need whereas a solution might still seem threatening to him. Try hearing his last statement as "please help me meet my needs" instead of an accusation. What might he be saying?

Nurse: You need to solve this dilemma, don't you Bill? You want to know you're vigilant and getting your son what he needs. And at the same time, you need to give your body a break. So you want what every father wants, to know you can relax and trust that your son will get good care.

Bill: Yeah. (Bill's whole body relaxes. He puts his head in his hands.) I've got to do all this myself. And it's hard.

Coach: I notice he's relaxing now. I'm betting you have a much better connection. He may be ready for some kind of solution. What would you suggest given what you know?

Nurse: Bill, your son's care is the most important thing to me. And I really want you to be healthy for him and for yourself.

Would you be willing to work something out with me so you can trust that we're watching him while you get some rest? Then we can work out these other issues.

Bill: Well. (Bill's eyes get red and watery.) Yeah. Thanks. That would help.

Nurse: Would you like to finish talking about your son's care now or would you rather schedule a time we can talk?

How did it work?

When the staff returned to their clinic to work with the family, confrontations continued but tended not to escalate. The staff preferred to handle them personally. The family noticed the improvement in relations and asked to delay transfer out of the department. Moreover, staff members who received training took their own initiative and personal time to brief the staff from the next department that would receive the family.

Reread the interaction. As you read it this time, underline the passages that illustrate how the Nurse used the ALIVE model to build rapport with Bill and uncover his needs. In the margin, make notes about how each step built rapport.

Then, turn the page to see what we thought.

Here's what we saw.

Assess your rapport	**Nurse:** If you're asking if I'm feeling good about this, then no, I'm not. When the Nurse checked in with her own feelings, she was gauging the rapport she had with her patient. And she found she was unhappy with it.
Listen for a call for help	**Coach:** Ok, you're solving his son's problems. What might Bill need? When the coach redirected the Nurse's attention to Bill rather than his son, he was reminding her to listen for a call for help about Bill.
Intend to connect	**Coach:** Why don't you try focusing on him a moment? Focusing on Bill is the first step in connecting.
Verify what's alive	**Nurse:** Bill, you look just exhausted to me. Are you feeling really tired? These, of course, are inquiries into Bill's feelings
Verify what's alive	**Nurse:** (to Bill) You look like you could use some kind of relief. The Nurse clarifies his needs before she moves on to solutions.

More of what we saw.

Assess your rapport	**Nurse:** OK, that hurt. I want to tell him that it wasn't my fault, that he can trust us. But I don't think he'll believe it. The Nurse revisits rapport and still finds she has more building to do.
Listen for a call for help	**Coach:** Try hearing his last statement as "please help me meet my needs" instead of an accusation. This is a clear reminder to listen for a call for help.
Intend to connect	**Coach:** What might he be saying? Curiosity is the foundation of an intention to connect.
Verify what's alive	**Nurse:** You need to solve this dilemma, don't you Bill? … trust that your son will get good care. Her whole statement is a verification of Bill's needs. She's identified the needs that would stop Bill from accepting the first strategy she wanted to propose—rest.
	Nurse: Bill, your son's care is the most important thing to me. And I really want you to be healthy for him and for yourself. She adds this step of underscoring that she wants Bill to get his needs met. This is often very effective once you have rapport.
Encourage a request that enriches life	**Nurse:** Would you like to finish talking about your son's care now, or would you rather schedule a time we can talk? Once they have rapport, she offers a solution.

Make it Last

The Three Levers of Lasting Change

You've seen ALIVE from end to end. This is a good time for you to check in with yourself. Your needs and your beliefs will guide your actions. Your actions will produce results. And you'll compare your results with your needs to decide how you want to invest in creating powerful experiences with patients over time.

Think back over what you've read and the work you've done. Assessing your rapport as a signal to use empathy. Listening to accusations and judgments as a call for help. Setting your intention to connect with patients. Verifying what they feel and need. And encouraging them to make a concrete request that will better meet their needs.

"You'll compare your results with your needs to decide how you want to invest in creating powerful experiences with patients over time."

Beliefs

What beliefs do you notice still stand in the way of creating powerful interactions with patients (Breaker Beliefs)? What beliefs have you developed that will aid you (Booster Beliefs)? And how can you reframe your Breaker Beliefs in other ways that support you?

For example, Sean has a Breaker Belief that he doesn't have time to discuss patients' feelings. He decides to reframe the belief by recognizing that feelings are a vital part of his patients' health. And he wants to show care for all aspects of his patients' health.

My Breaker Beliefs

1. _____

2. _____

3. _____

4. _____

5. _____

   _____

My Booster Beliefs

1. _____

2. _____

3. _____

4. _____

5. _____

   _____

Other ways I can think of my Breaker Beliefs so that they support me.

1. _____

2. _____

3. _____

4. _____

5. _____

   _____

Personal practices

We've recommended a set of practices that will help you focus your attention where you're more likely to get what you want. What are some things you can do that will support you in putting the skills to use? Here are some examples we like:

∴ Get a "learning partner," someone you can talk to about what you're doing and can practice the skills with you

∴ Make commitments to yourself or others about how you'll learn or practice these skills

∴ Put up reminders to yourself about your goals for the day or week or month

∴ Supply yourself with reading and listening material that reinforces the skills and attitudes you want to adopt

"By prizing heartfulness above faultlessness, we may reap more from our effort because we're more likely to be changed by it."

Sharon Salzberg

What examples are appealing to you:

1. _____

2. _____

3. _____

4. _____

5. _____

_____

_____

Organizational Environment

Look around your organization. What do you notice that helps you create powerful interactions or that undermines you?

What would you like to encourage your organization to do? Here are some places to look:

Building policies or strategies that support patients or revising policies that show disregard for them.

1. _____

2. _____

3. _____

Creating signage that reminds you to show support for patients or revising décor that doesn't.

1. _____

2. _____

3. _____

Increasing the topics you handle in internal meetings that foster powerful relationships with patients (for example, sharing stories of great encounters with patients or great encounters the staff has had as customers of any business) or decreasing the time you spend on topics that don't contribute to powerful relationships with patients.

1. _____

2. _____

3. _____

Your Action Plan

Given what you've learned, what will you do to improve your organization's relationships with patients? Be as specific as you can. A specific goal will have all the elements of good request: it can be measured, has a timeline, is achievable (not solving world hunger next week), and yields concrete results.

As an example, Shawn might plan within a week to ask his manager if she'd be willing to put $30 of the department budget toward posting signs behind the lobby counter that remind staff to take time to show empathy to patients making appointments.

What I'll do	When I'll get it done
1. _____	____/____/____
2. _____	____/____/____
3. _____	____/____/____
4. _____	____/____/____
5. _____	____/____/____
6. _____	____/____/____

Taking a Compassionate Stand

In Section One, we defined empathy as a respectful understanding of another person's reality. We described the goal for empathy skills

∴ enable healers to create a heartfelt connection with patients—so each has the experience of being listened to respectfully and having their needs taken seriously.

And we introduced the ALIVE process for giving active empathy to patients.

In Section Two, we went deeply into the skills covered in the last two steps of the ALIVE process:

∴ **Verify what's alive** and

∴ **Encourage a request that enriches life.**

We saw that these two steps encompass four skills:

1. Helping your patients separate their observations from their judgments,
2. Helping them identify their feelings,
3. Uncovering their needs, and
4. Helping them form requests to meet those needs.

That's the ALIVE process for giving empathy to others.

But what about you? What about getting your needs met?

If you're following the ALIVE process, you're already experiencing some pay off. You're taking patients' comments less personally. You're having encounters that are more gratifying. You're using skills that reinforce your ability to contribute and create good outcomes for patients.

You likely also have a sense that there's more. You're giving a lot of empathy and you'd like to get more empathy in return. You know your encounters could go even better if you could garner the same kind of compassion for your needs and views that you offer to your patients.

We opened this conversation in Section One by talking about developing a mutual desire to give from the heart. So let's take up the flip side of giving empathy; namely, speaking honestly, or taking a compassionate stand for yourself.

We'll use the same overall process:

Assess your rapport

Listen for a call for help

Intend to connect

Verify what's alive

Encourage a request that enriches life

The first three steps—assess your rapport, listen for a call for help, and intend to connect—set the stage for a strong connection.

The fourth step—verify what's alive—is the actual process of connecting with your patient or other staff members.

In the fifth step—encourage a request—you generate strategies that meet your needs as well as the needs of your patient and your organization.

Let's begin by imagining that you want to talk to a patient or your peers about something that's left you unhappy.

Suppose a patient has put a reclining chair in front of the emergency kit in a patient room and no other staff member has asked them to move it. So you see two discussions before you.

1. You want to let your patient know you think the chair is in an unsafe place.

2. And you want to confront your fellow staff members about letting your patient leave the chair there.

We'll take a brief look how each of the steps applies to speaking honestly. Then we'll take the final two steps in depth as we did in Section Two.

Assess your rapport

rapport [ra·páwr], noun, *an easy relationship people enjoy based on mutual trust, and a sense that they understand each other's concerns.*

If you recall how we defined rapport in the previous Section, you'll notice that it's different from friendship. It's a sense of trust and understanding in the moment.

Chances are, if you'd like your patient to behave differently, you don't share a common understanding of each other's concerns. And even if you are friends with your fellow staff members, you likely anticipate that you'll be at odds over this issue.

Remember that an uneasy feeling is a signal, not to lay back or tip-toe, but to engage in an exchange of empathy.

You can use ALIVE to do just that.

Listen for a call for help

If you're like most people, as you imagine preparing for these conversations, you *brace* yourself. You ask yourself if you think you can win these arguments you anticipate. You check in with yourself to see *who's right*. And you do a mental calculation of *who has the most power*.

You can take this thinking into your confrontations. And you'll likely win this one. After all, you have authority, hospital policy, and the patient's safety on your side.

But what about those times you don't? What about the times you're the most junior person on the team? Or you have a conviction that others may not readily share? **Even in those cases, you can be powerful, there's a way to take a stand.**

It starts with you recognizing your internal bracing as a loss of rapport and a call for help. You can listen to your internal judgments and uncover your own needs that are going unmet. Your need to contribute to your patient's well-being. Your need to experience as much ease and harmony as possible in your workplace.

Just like your patients, you are always **either showing gratitude or asking for help**.

So your next step is to ask yourself, **"How can I hear my own judgments as my request for help?"** There's no need to resist your internal judgments. They serve you.

Simply, shift the way you listen to them. Recognize your unmet needs spoken through your judgments. And you'll open up a whole new line of interaction.

Intend to connect

Normally, when we're preparing for discussions like these, we're figuring out how to win, or at least not lose. *That intention subconsciously triggers defensiveness in other people.* And their defensiveness will make it harder, not easier, for you to get what you need.

I don't suggest that you abandon your point. Just remind yourself that you can get what you need without anyone else being wrong or weaker than you are. You can advocate vigorously for your needs without worrying about whom the world would call *right* or who's *higher in the pecking order*.

Again, as when you were listening with empathy, the first three steps of the ALIVE model can be done in seconds or less. It's a quick internal check followed by a couple of shifts in perspective—assess your rapport, listen to your judgments as a call for help, intend to connect. Together they prepare you mentally to engage effectively with your patient or your co-workers.

Focusing on What's Alive in You

1. Report your observations, what you see, hear, or sense that meets your needs or doesn't.

2. Say how you feel when you observe these actions

3. Identify which of your needs are behind your feelings.

Verify what's alive

Recall that **our goal is to arrive at a mutual desire to give from the heart.** Not to dominate. Not to win. Just to tell others what you need. To listen to their needs, in turn. And to form strategies that work for both of you.

We nurture this mutual desire by focusing our attention on what's alive in us, what we feel and what we need. That's a three-step process.

Encourage a request that enriches life

We follow the three steps immediately by suggesting a specific request that might better meet our needs. For example, "Would you be willing to tell me what you just heard?" if you need understanding most at the moment.

This is the flip side of being open to those four aspects of your patient's experience. **You connect by being clear about what you observe, feel, need, and what actions would better meet your needs and the needs of your organization.**

The skills are the steps in a dance that's familiar to you. As we express what's alive in ourselves and attend to what's alive in our patients, back and forth, we uncover our humanity. What arises is a mutual desire to give from the heart.

We'll explore in the following units this model of expressing yourself clearly and honestly.

But first, we need to take into account your position in your organization and the way your natural authority inflects your communication.

...Because it's our policy

Language that gets in the way of compassion

We're developing a process of communicating that underscores human connection, the connection between a staff member and other staff members or patients. That kind of language tends to foster a mutual desire to give from the heart.

In contrast, bureaucratic language obscures the connection between a person and his actions or desires. By clouding the speaker's humanity, it tends to trigger defensiveness in others.

You and your sweet desires

Unfortunately, our language teaches us to separate ourselves from our desires, even those we hold most dear. Imagine a colleague approaches you on the job. Write your gut reaction to hearing each of the following phrases they might say to you.

Example 1

I need some rest.

When I hear this phrase from a co-worker, I feel

_____

_____

_____

I *deserve* a break.

When I hear this phrase from a co-worker, I feel

_____

_____

_____

Example 2:

I'm afraid for the patient's safety.

When I hear this phrase from a co-worker, I feel

_____

_____

_____

It's our *policy*.

When I hear this phrase from a co-worker, I feel

_____

_____

_____

Example 3:

I need help at the top of the shift and I'm upset about the amount of work I end up doing when you come in at quarter after.

When I hear this phrase from a co-worker, I feel

_____

_____

_____

You *have to* start showing up on time.

When I hear this phrase from a co-worker, I feel

_____

_____

_____

Example 4:

I'd like to have confidence that you'll do your part, including folding the sheets.

When I hear this phrase from a co-worker, I feel

_____

_____

After all I do around here, you can't even fold the sheets like you're *supposed* to.

When I hear this phrase from a co-worker, I feel

_____

_____

The statements on the right appear to be more to the point because they're briefer. But in their brevity, **they obscure the connection between the speaker and his convictions,** his feelings, his needs. And **by clouding that connection, they threaten the connection between the speaker and the listener,** you and your patient or co-worker.

I want... I feel... I need...
Statements that start with these phrases are naturally powerful. They're indisputable. I can challenge whether you *deserve* a break but I simply accept that you *want* one. These phrases do a better job of setting the stage for connection because they reveal my humanity. And they're more accurate. I don't *have to* start showing up on time whether or not you're angry when I show up after my shift has begun.

Translating "Have to, Must, and Should" to "Choose to"

Column 1	Column 2	Column 3
_____	1. _____	_____
	_____	_____
_____	2. _____	_____
	_____	_____
_____	3. _____	_____
	_____	_____

Here's a reminder of the natural autonomy each of us enjoys—patients and caregivers alike. Start by listing three things you do because you have to. These can come from your job or from other parts of your life. List them as 1, 2, and 3 in Column 2 above.

Second, acknowledge that you have a choice. **The choice may be difficult or painful, but you disable yourself when you ignore that you have it.** To remind yourself of your autonomy, your power of choice, use Column 1 to write "I choose to" before each thing you do in Column 2.

Finally, look at each activity you've listed, 1 through 3. Consider your intention behind each thing you do. What do you ultimately want? Then, in Column 3, write "because I want" and finish the phrase by listing what you hope to get by doing whatever it is you do.

When you're done, you'll end up with three statements that look something like this:

I choose to	drive 45 minutes to work every day	Because I want to keep my house and job

Once you've changed your "have tos" into "choose tos" there are a number of questions you can ask yourself

1. Are the things you want in Column 3 worth doing the actions you've listed in Column 2?

2. Are the actions you've listed in Column 2 the way you'd prefer to get what you want in Column 3?

3. Are the motivations you've listed in Column 3 the kinds of things you'd like to have driving your decisions? Have you listed, for instance, "People expect me to", or "I'd feel guilty if I didn't"? If you have, you might ask yourself how you enjoy letting other people's opinions drive your actions.

Whatever conclusions you come to, you'll be clearer in your communications when you remember that you are like your patients in this respect: **whatever you do, you do to meet your own needs**. Even when our society teaches us to say we're doing it because we must, it's our job, or it's policy, we always do what we do to meet our own needs.

Do You See What I See?

Making clear OBSERVATIONS and owning your judgments

Suppose you want to express yourself honestly to a patient or co-worker. The first step is to be clear about what you're seeing, hearing, and sensing that affects your well-being.

To do that, you'll want to separate your judgments from your evaluations. Not become objective. Just clarify your observations and own the judgments you make regarding what you observe.

"When you mix observations and evaluations or judgments, the people you're talking to will tend to hear criticism. And you'll be less likely to get what you want."

When you mix observations and evaluations or judgments, the people you're talking to will tend to hear criticism. And you'll be less likely to get what you want.

I was reminded of the problems with mixing observations and judgments while working with a medical unit on alleviating complaints. They wanted training on setting boundaries and implementing a no-tolerance policy (no loud or abusive language). The manager asked me how her staff could warn each other about patients who were rude and aggressive without labeling the patients as rude and aggressive.

Then she frowned at the irony of her own request.

If there is a way to label people without labeling them, I don't know it.

The solution is not to stop judging. How could you do that? Rather, it's to own your judgments and become aware of the observations that lead you to your judgments.

Put yourself in your co-worker's place. Which of the following two reports would be more helpful for you?

Mr. Hsieh is unpredictable and aggressive.

OR...

When I responded to the call button, Mr Hsieh raised his voice, stepped very close to me, and asked me why the medication was late last night. His behavior seems very aggressive to me.

No matter which report you received you'd need more information to create a good experience with Mr. Hsieh. You'd want to understand, for example, what was driving his concern about the timing of the medication.

But the second report gives you a lot more to go on. And empathy skills, as you've seen, can help you collect the remaining information you need.

Notice also that you don't have to stop judging people. ALIVE simply suggests that you'll have better interactions and outcomes when you separate your observations from your evaluations.

As when you are listening with empathy, there are two ways you can clarify your observations. You can

∴ clarify the actions you've observed that are at the source of your judgments

∴ clarify the specific time and context of observations rather than expressing them as generalizations

When you separate your interpretations from your observations, you'll be less likely to pass your judgments on to your co-workers. And your comments will be easier for your patients to listen to as well. In the examples that follow, put yourself in the place of the listener. Which comment would you be most receptive to?

Example #1

1st caregiver: When you create a health hazard like that....

2nd caregiver: When the chair is between the emergency kit and the bed...

Example #2

1st caregiver: It's irresponsible to come in late like this.

2nd caregiver: When I see you come in twenty minutes after your shift has started, I think you're irresponsible.

Example #3

1st caregiver: You're just dangerous with a needle.

2nd caregiver: When I see you try for a vein for a third time in one place, I think it's dangerous.

Your intention isn't to sugar-coat everything you say. We don't pretend that there's a way to phrase everything that leaves the listener happy you spoke.

But when you make clear observations and take responsibility for your judgments, other people will be more likely to hear the message you intend.

You'll help yourself even more by focusing on and identifying the needs that lie beneath your judgments. You might want to take a look back at Unit Seven in Section Two for a reminder.

Rewrite these statements to make clear what you've seen or heard that leads to your evaluation.

1. You're always in such a rush.

   _____

   _____

2. When it comes to room changes, you guys aren't doing your jobs.

   _____

   _____

3. There's no way he's going to stay on that treatment schedule.

   _____

   _____

4. He doesn't take care of his body.

   _____

   _____

Here are some answers we liked.

1. You're always in such a rush.
   We haven't spent more than 5 minutes on a shift report any night this week.

2. When it comes to room changes, you guys aren't doing your jobs.
   When patients tell me they had no warning they might need to move, I think you aren't doing your job.

3. There's no way he's going to stay on that treatment schedule.
   I don't think there's any way he's going to stay on that treatment schedule.

4. He doesn't take care of his body.
   He's twenty pounds overweight and he was eating a candy bar when he came in here.

The answers I give for #'s 2 and 3 are only subtly different from the original phrasing. In each of the exercises, the caregiver makes a proclamation about another person— "You guys aren't…" or "There's no way he's going to…" I recommend you rephrase the statement to show that the speaker is aware he's stating an opinion—"I think you aren't" and "I don't think there's any way…"

In both of these cases, you may be concerned that the listener won't enjoy the opinion the speaker expresses. I agree with you. I wouldn't enjoy hearing those comments directed at me. But again, our objective is to be honest and accurate, not to pretend we don't have judgments.

If you're looking for a more effective way to work through your own judgments, look back at Unit Seven in Section Two where we talked about stating the needs beneath judgments.

In your life

Think of two judgments or generalizations you are often tempted to make. Write down a statement you might make to help clarify *the actions you've observed* that are at the source of your judgments or *the specific time and context of observations* that you might otherwise express as a generalization.

1. Judgment or generalization you are tempted to make

_____

_____

_____

Statement you could make to clarify the observation

_____

_____

_____

2. Judgment or generalization you are tempted to make

_____

_____

_____

Statement you could make to clarify the observation

_____

_____

_____

How I feel...

Expressing your FEELINGS honestly

The second step in the process of verifying what's alive in you is clarifying the feelings that your observations have triggered.

Staff members are often wary of letting patients know how they feel. You may be concerned that revealing your fears will make you appear weak. But my experience is that your strength comes from your conviction to meet your own needs and help others meet theirs. Not from your lack of fear.

"Your strength comes from your conviction to meet your own needs and help others meet theirs."

Other times, we're afraid that patients will be upset because they want us to focus on them, not ourselves. In our training, though, we see that patients are interested in anything that affects their experience of care. Your feelings are fair game as long as they're relevant to your patients' experience. I learned the power of expressing feelings during a training program for a group of nurses. We were working on an encounter between a young man and a female nurse.

She had been listening and showing real empathy for several minutes. No matter how she identified what the man was feeling and what he needed, his anger never dissipated.

Finally, she turned to tell me she was frustrated and she wished she could let him know. When I suggested that she do that, she said, "I'm doing what I know how to do. And I don't see any signs that you're getting what you want. I am so frustrated!" To which he responded, "Well, now you know how I feel!"

It broke the conversation open and they were finally able to uncover his great hesitancy to trust the staff. He said he hadn't heard anyone talk to him in a way he believed was honest until she admitted her frustration.

Another time we were working with a group of senior nurses. I was interacting with an Asian man who had limited English and a reputation for being abrupt and unpredictable.

During the interaction, the man moved suddenly close to me and raised his hands and his voice. I stepped back and said, "I really want to help. When you step in close like that, I get a bit scared and it's harder for me to focus on helping." He stepped right back and lowered his voice.

One of the supervising nurses rushed up to me after the demonstration and said, "Oh that was wonderful, especially when you said you were scared. If only our doctors in the ER could do that, it would really help them."

My goal isn't to give you a magic phrase that will open up conversations. It's to encourage you to stay present in your conversations, listen with empathy, speak the truth, and trust that compassion will manifest.

All the recommendations I gave you in Section Two for helping your patient's express their feelings apply to you as well.

In particular, there's nothing wrong with telling people what you think. Just be clear.

To express your thinking, talk about your thoughts. When you want to express your feelings, use a straightforward language of emotions.

I feel frustrated.

NOT,

I feel threatened.

Threatened isn't a feeling; it's my belief about what you are trying to do to me (threaten me).

and NOT,

I feel that you're being unresponsive.

You're being unresponsive is a judgment I have about how you're acting. And I'd want to disclose what I see that leads me to that judgment.

and NOT,

I feel incompetent.

Incompetent is a judgment I have of myself. And if I were going to talk that way to myself, I'd want to remind myself what I'm observing that leads me to that judgment.

But simply,

I feel scared, frustrated, or irritated (if I'm not getting my needs met).

Or

I feel happy, thrilled, or gratified (if I am getting my needs met).

Again, to identify your feelings, you just listen internally for a gut reaction. That usually produces a feeling word—sad, mad, glad, or afraid.

How you doin'?

Take on the role of the caregiver in the examples below. Rewrite the statement to clearly express how you feel.

Make the emotions behind these statements clear.

117

1. **I feel like he doesn't listen to me**

Rewrite:_____

_____

2. **I feel unimportant around here.**

Rewrite:_____

_____

3. **I feel you really see me and appreciate me.**

Rewrite:_____

_____

4. **I feel invisible.**

Rewrite:_____

_____

Here are some answers we liked.

1. I feel like he doesn't listen to me

Rewrite: **I get angry when he starts talking before I've finished.**

2. I feel unimportant around here.

Rewrite: **I'm frustrated that I haven't received an invitation for the past three staff meetings.**

3. I feel you really see me and appreciate me.

Rewrite: **I'm so proud to get this certificate.**

4. I feel invisible.

Rewrite: **I'm pretty comfortable. I don't really have to stretch myself.**

This last answer may strike you as unlikely. It might help to imagine two people—Bob and Eric—in different circumstances. Bob is happy he's invisible and Eric is resentful. What are the different circumstances, attitudes, and needs that lead Bob and Eric to their different feelings about seeming invisible?

All I really need

The key to better experiences

By now you know that needs are the core of empathy. Let me boil it down to three axioms:

1. Each of us is the source of our own thoughts and needs, and those in turn cause our feelings.

2. We have better experiences to the extent that we get our needs met. Hence, we're highly motivated to get our needs met. Everything we do, in fact, we do to meet our needs.

3. We're more likely to get out needs met when a) we're clear about what they are, and b) we demonstrate that we have a stake in other people getting their needs met as well.

You can look back at Unit Seven of Section Two for a review of needs. There you'll find discussions and exercises that explain

∴   The key misunderstanding about why we feel what we feel: we mistakenly believe that others are responsible for our feelings

∴   The four ways you can listen to someone else's judgment, and why you'll be more effective when you hear it as a call for help

∴   The difference between needs (that are universal) and strategies (that are particular to people)

∴   How to translate accusations and judgments into a language of needs.

∴   A list of universal needs

∴   The gift of victim language: it reveals needs, and

121

∴ when to focus on feelings with a patient (when you're unsure how she feels) and when to focus on needs (when feelings are already clear)

In this unit, we'll talk over the problems surrounding needs that most often plague caregivers.

You can use the skills this way, but I don't recommend it

If you've begun to put these skills to use, you've noticed that you can burn yourself out really quickly.

There are three ways that caregivers can burn themselves in regards to their needs.

1. You can come to see yourself as responsible for other people's experience rather than responsive to them,

2. You can ignore your own needs, and

3. You can express your needs in ways that lead others to respond with resistance rather than empathy.

We'll talk through each problem in turn and suggest simple solutions for you.

Be responsive to others, but don't take responsibility for their feelings

Of course, you want to take care of your patients. You want to support your co-workers. At the same time, you need to let their experience be theirs. Otherwise, you take on the responsibility of *making them happy* which we know you can't deliver on.

Here's an example of a caregiver taking on responsibility for his patient's experience.

Patient: I'm such a burden to my family.

Caregiver: No, no, you're doing the best you can. I'm sure they don't think you're any trouble at all.

Instead, the caregiver can take himself out of the picture and simply be present to the patient's concerns.

Caregiver: You'd really like some way of helping your loved ones through this.

Below, again the caregiver takes on responsibility for her co-worker's experience.

Co-worker: I don't see why I always have to deal with Mr. Bunsen. Can't anyone else handle him?

Caregiver: They really do push you too hard, don't they? Can't they see you already have enough on your plate?

Instead, she can simply be responsive to her co-worker, like this.

Caregiver: You'd really like a break, huh?

"When I learned to meet my thinking as a friend, I noticed that I could meet every human as a friend."

Byron Katie
Loving What Is

Take responsibility for your patients' and co-workers' happiness and you'll begin to see them as burdens. And your job will leave you exhausted.

Acknowledge the needs of others, but don't ignore your own needs

Another way to burn out helping others is to pay attention **only to the last half of the needs-based skills.** Focus on helping other people identify their needs. Negotiate solutions that help them get their needs met while ignoring yours.

Where does that leave you? Suffering.

I often see caregivers twist *caring* into a denial of their own needs in order to attend to the needs of other sufferers.

Follow this path, and you'll end up resenting your patients and resenting your job. **It's this kind of burn out that leads caregivers to judge their patients and label them needy, dependent, or ungrateful.** Or to say, even to yourself, "you know what, that's your problem."

The solution isn't to resist your judgments. It's to listen to them, hear your own call for help, and **admit your needs.**

Below you'll see the internal dialogue for two caregivers. You'll first see their judgments. Then, you'll see how they've accepted those judgments and translated them into statements of their own needs.

"Our culture is designed to make women keenly aware of what others want, at the expense of an awareness of their own needs."

Kelly Bryson

Example #1

Judgment: The patient in 301 wants me in his room constantly. What's wrong with him that he can't be alone for a few minutes?

Needs: When I see the kind of pain my patients are in, it's hard for me to think about myself. I could really use some attention, someone interested in me for a little bit.

Example #2

Judgment: How can she blame me for that outcome? I told her about the risks. She's just a gold-digger.

Needs: It's frightening to hear a patient so unhappy and blaming me. I'd rather we were working together to decide what to do next. And I could use just a little recognition for the care I took and the time I spent with her.

Express your needs clearly, you'll be more likely to get empathy rather than resistance

Sacrifice and bearing up have become part and parcel of our concept of a caregiver. We're afraid to admit we have needs and afraid to ask plainly for help. The requests that do finally surface often come out sideways, as unimpeachable cases we've built to justify our needs.

Unfortunately, rather than evoking empathy, the cases we build usually bring out resistance. And the rejection we experience when others hear our case only confirms for us that they don't care about our needs.

Here's an example of how a caregiver can strip away her own "legal case" to reveal the need beneath it:

Legal Case: You said you'd only need me an extra hour or so. Well it's three o'clock, isn't it? I not only took the extra time, I took Bill's patients while he was down in radiology, for goodness knows what. I feel like an orderly. You know I haven't sat down all day. And my lunch is still in the bag. There's no way I'm going to be eating it in the break room for dinner.

Needs: I've had a busy day. I'm exhausted. I'd like to go home now.

After each statement, identify the problem the caregiver is having with stating his or her needs:

∴ Being responsible instead of responsive

∴ Expressing needs as judgments, or

∴ Building a legal case.

Then rewrite the statement to make the caregiver's needs clear and to make it clear that the caregiver and patient are each responsible for his or her own experience.

1. Oh you poor thing, your family had no call to treat you that way.

❑ Being responsible instead of responsive	❑ Expressing needs as judgments	❑ Building a legal case

Your Rewrite:

_____

_____

2. Would you please get back inside and get to work. We have two therapists out today and I'm taking up the slack. You wouldn't believe the stack of paperwork I have to do before I go home. I have three complaints to write up. And you two have time for a smoke.

❑ Being responsible instead of responsive	❑ Expressing needs as judgments	❑ Building a legal case

Your Rewrite:

_____

_____

_____

3. Man, are you on an ego trip or what? I swear you give me cases just to show you can.

❑ Being responsible instead of responsive	❑ Expressing needs as judgments	❑ Building a legal case

Your Rewrite:

_____

_____

_____

4. What does she think; she's the only patient I have? She's so demanding!

☐ Being responsible instead of responsive	☐ Expressing needs as judgments	☐ Building a legal case

Your Rewrite:

_____

_____

_____

5. What do you think I am: food service, a janitor, and housekeeping? I have to do everything around here. I wasn't trained for this and I didn't sign up for this. I'm so underutilized. Why don't you give me the work you hired me for?

☐ Being responsible instead of responsive	☐ Expressing needs as judgments	☐ Building a legal case

Your Rewrite:

_____

_____

_____

_____

6. I'm sorry I'm so late. I can see why that makes you so mad.

☐ Being responsible instead of responsive	☐ Expressing needs as judgments	☐ Building a legal case

Your Rewrite:

_____

_____

_____

Here are some answers we liked.

1. Oh you poor thing, your family had no call to treat you that way.

☑ Being responsible instead of responsive	❑ Expressing needs as judgments	❑ Building a legal case

Your Rewrite: **You sound pretty desolate, like you could use some comfort and company.**

2. Would you two please get back inside and get to work. We have two therapists out today and I'm taking up the slack. You wouldn't believe the stack of paperwork I have to do before I go home. I have three complaints to write up. And you two have time for smoke.

❑ Being responsible instead of responsive	❑ Expressing needs as judgments	☑ Building a legal case

Your Rewrite: **I'm so harried. I could really use some support.**

3. Man, are you on an ego trip or what? I swear you give me cases just to show you can.

❑ Being responsible instead of responsive	☑ Expressing needs as judgments	❑ Building a legal case

Your Rewrite: **I'd like to help you out. Frankly, what I really need right now is some sleep.**

4. What does she think; she's the only patient I have? She's so demanding!

☐ Being responsible instead of responsive	☑ Expressing needs as judgments	☐ Building a legal case

Your Rewrite: **I could use some understanding for how busy I am and some credit for how much I do for her.**

5. What do you think I am: food service, a janitor, and housekeeping? I have to do everything around here. I wasn't trained for this and I didn't sign up for this. I'm so underutilized. Why don't you give me the work you hired me for?

☐ Being responsible instead of responsive	☐ Expressing needs as judgments	☑ Building a legal case

Your Rewrite: **I need to do work that's more meaningful to me.**

6. I'm sorry I'm so late. I can see why that makes you so mad.

☑ Being responsible instead of responsive	☐ Expressing needs as judgments	☐ Building a legal case

Your Rewrite: **You'd like some consideration for the value of your time.**

Let's get real

List three instances you see when caregivers have difficulty stating their needs. They could be times that a caregiver takes responsibility for another person's feelings, when she ignores her own needs and they come out as criticisms, or when he makes a case instead of stating a need. Follow each instance with a clear statement of the caregiver's needs.

1. How you see your self or other caregivers having trouble stating their needs

_____

_____

Statement you could make to clarify needs

_____

_____

2. How you see your self or other caregivers having trouble stating their needs

_____

_____

Statement you could make to clarify needs

_____

_____

3. How you see your self or other caregivers having trouble stating their needs

_____

_____

Statement you could make to clarify needs

_____

_____

Would you be willing to...

Encouraging REQUESTS that enrich life

The previous three units of this Section covered the heart of the ALIVE model, **V**erify what's alive. We began by separating your observations from your judgments. Then you named your feelings. Finally, we talked about expressing your needs in ways that will likely get you what you want.

In this unit, we'll discuss the final step of the ALIVE model, Encourage a request that enriches life. For a review of requests, you can look back at Unit Eight of Section Two. There you'll find discussions about the importance of

demand
[di·mánd], noun,
a request that is difficult to deny

∴ verifying needs before you form requests,

∴ making implied requests explicit, and

∴ forming requests that are specific enough to work.

The framework we provide for making well-formed requests for patients also applies to the requests you make to meet your own needs.

In this unit, we'll discuss challenges that face caregivers who are making requests.

1. The difference between requests and demands

2. What to do when someone says "no" to a request you think is important

3. Diffusing requests that sound like demands

4. Making requests of people who you see as having more power or seniority

Smile when you say that...

In our training programs, when we ask how you can tell a request from a demand, people most often say that a request is spoken in a different tone of voice, or it's preceded by a "please".

Reflect a moment and you'll realize this isn't it. Very simply, the difference between a request and a demand is whether the listener can feel free to say "no" or he's afraid his "no" will be punished.

Here's how that might look in action:

Caregiver: I need you to prep Mr. Bodi for his GI today.

Co-worker: He's not my patient. Can you get Rachel to do it?

The co-worker has said "no". The caregiver's next response will determine whether your co-worker perceives the original request as a demand. If she thinks she's being punished, she'll hear the original request as a demand. Here are some examples:

Punishing the co-worker with a judgment:

Caregiver: I can't believe how stingy you are with your time.

Punishing the co-worker with guilt:

Caregiver: You really aren't a team player are you?

Threatening your co-worker with your power:

Caregiver: If I say he's your patient, he's your patient. Do you understand?

If, on the other hand, the caregiver shows empathy, the co-worker will believe she can say no and she'll hear the original request as authentic.

Caregiver: Are you already feeling pretty overwhelmed today?

Why this is important to you

Because when you try to force your co-worker to say "yes," they'll perceive you as making a demand. And none of us likes to honor demands. We think we're giving in to bullying.

We all prize our autonomy, our freedom to choose. When your patients or co-workers hear your request as a demand, their reflex will be to resist. Even if you're senior or seen as more powerful, we'll tend to subvert what you want even as we acquiesce to you.

That's going to leave you in a pincer when you have a request that's important to you. You'll want to be as persuasive as possible without inviting resistance, backlash, and subterfuge.

Don't stop at "no"

Of course, there are times you'll want to make demands. Often, especially in medical emergencies, you'll be unwilling to debate the merits of your requests.

But what about the other times—when you're making requests of a co-worker or someone senior, when you know your patient is about to walk out the door and you want them to continue following your recommendations even after you're out of earshot? How can you be most effective, when their first reaction is to say no?

How to Work Effectively with "No"

1. Acknowledge the no, so you know where you stand.

2. Give the speaker empathy; explore the good reasons she has for saying "no".

3. Make another request taking into account what you've learned about her needs.

Making requests instead of demands doesn't mean giving up power. You can redouble your effectiveness in making requests by using the three step process in the box at the left.

When you think about it, this is no different from the framework we've been working through. You simply take the "no" as a sign of a lack of rapport, and continue with the model. Look back at the case study at the end of Section Two and you'll see this process in action. A nurse is talking to Bill, a disgruntled father who doesn't seem to appreciate the requests that the nurse is drawing out. Early in the encounter, the nurse guesses that Bill really needs a rest but anticipates his no.

Nurse: (to the coach) I want to tell him that I can find a place for him to sleep but my suggestions haven't seemed to make him very happy so far.

She gives Bill empathy and draws out additional needs.

Nurse: You need to solve this dilemma, don't you Bill? You want to know you're being a good father and vigilant. And at the same time, you need to give your body a break. So you want what every father wants, to know you can relax and trust that your son will get good care.

After she's drawn out his need to feel trust, she returns to the suggestion of rest and incorporates her new insights.

Nurse: Bill, your son's care is the most important thing to me. And I really want you to be healthy for him and for yourself [letting him know she wants him to get his needs met]. Would you be willing to work something out with me so you can trust that we're watching your son while you get some rest? Then we can work out these other issues.

It's this request that Bill agrees to.

Your turn

After each exchange, write a question that can help the caregiver uncover the need that leads the other speaker to say no.

Example #1

Caregiver: We need to schedule you for another round of treatments.

Patient: You can schedule what you want, but I'm not coming in for this again.

Caregiver: _____

Example #2

Caregiver: I need the results of Mrs. Jacob's tests by 1:00.

Co-worker: That's really your problem isn't it?

Caregiver: _____

Example #3

Caregiver: Would you like a referral to an agency that can help with that?

Patient: That really isn't any of your business.

Caregiver: _____

Example #4

Caregiver: I thought we'd just keep her another day for observation.

Co-worker: You have my orders. I expect you to carry them out.

Caregiver: _____

Here are some answers we liked:

Example #1

Caregiver: We need to schedule you for another round of treatments.

Patient: You can schedule what you want, but I'm not coming in for this again.

Caregiver: Are you feeling discouraged and looking for something you can do that would give you more of a sense of hope?

Example #2

Caregiver: I need the results of Mrs. Jacob's tests by 1:00.

Co-worker: That's really your problems isn't it?

Caregiver: You're pretty swamped, huh? You need some time to dig yourself out?

Example #3

Caregiver: Would you like a referral to an agency that can help with that?

Patient: That really isn't any of your business.

Caregiver: You'd like some privacy on this issue?

Example #4

Caregiver: I thought we'd just keep her another day for observation.

Co-worker: You have my orders. I expect you to carry them out.

Caregiver: You'd like some sign from me that I respect your authority?

An imbalance of Power

You don't get cooperation from other people because you can demand it. Other people contribute to you because they are clear how they get what they need in the process.

Any staff member who's spent time in a healthcare organization can describe an intricate lattice of power relationships. Patients are less powerful than staff unless they're loud, or friends of patrons, or members of some protected class. Doctors are more powerful than nurses except in areas where the nurses are more experienced, or better connected, or have a closer relationship with the patient.

In fact, a common training question from new hires is "how do I find my voice"? Which translates roughly into "how do I talk to people before I figure out who I have to listen to and who has to listen to me?" Healthcare organizations, in other words, tend to produce interactions in which people are ready to hear demands and push back.

"Power With," not "Power Over"

The ALIVE process isn't based on having power over another person. Many people will experience that as a great strength. You get your needs out on the table. You help your co-worker lay his needs out as well. And together the two of you look for solutions that satisfy you both.

So power differences don't play a role in the ALIVE model. You don't get cooperation from other people because you can demand it. Other people contribute to you because they see your humanity and an opportunity for the gratification that comes from contributing. And because they are clear how they get what they need in the process.

Still, some in your organization have more power—formal and informal—than others. There's a way to work more effectively in each of those situations.

When you're "one up"

A supervisor is talking to a direct report. She wants him to take on extra work but only if he would do it with commitment.

"Only strength can cooperate."

Dwight D. Eisenhower

She makes a request, "I'd like you to head up this project." He says, "Yeah, sure." Now, the supervisor is afraid that he's taken her request as a demand and that he'll give the project half-hearted attention. She can monitor him closely, wait for signs of failure, and have another talk. Or she can take full accountability for the clarity of her communications, right now.

She starts with a request that will reveal whether she has the clarity she wants.

Supervisor: Listen, before we agree, can you tell me what you just heard me say?

Subordinate: Yeah, you said I've got this new project to do.

Her intuition is right. They don't understand each other. And she has a sense that telling him he's wrong isn't going to increase their rapport and further her goal. So she makes another request still focused on fostering clear communications.

Supervisor: Thanks for telling me what you heard. I wasn't as clear as I wanted to be. Can you suggest how I can ask you about this project so that it wouldn't sound like an assignment?

She works on the immediate need—a way of communicating so they understand each other. When she's satisfied that need, she'll go back to clarify her intentions for the project. The key is staying in the moment, handling the challenges one at a time: clarifying her intentions first, and then clarifying his decision.

Getting accountable for your own clarity

After each exchange, write a statement or question that would help the caregiver get the clarity he or she wants.

Example #1

Caregiver: I don't see that we're doing any good at this point. I'd like you to consider stopping the protocol.

Family member: You're the expert.

Caregiver: _____

Example #2

Caregiver: I'd like you to ask my opinion before you make decisions like that.

Supervisor: You really want to take that tone of voice with me?

Caregiver: _____

Here are some responses that I believe will help you meet your needs:

Example #1

Caregiver: I don't see that we're doing any good at this point. I'd like you to consider stopping the protocol.

Family member: You're the expert.

Caregiver: **Before you decide, would you be willing to tell me what you heard me advising you to do?**

In this case, the caregiver want to know that the family member heard her suggest that he "*consider* stopping the protocol", not just that she suggested that he stop the protocol.

Example #2

Caregiver: I'd like you to ask my opinion before you make decisions like that.

Supervisor: You really want to take that tone of voice with me?

Caregiver: **How can I phrase that so it sounds like a request and not like I'm trying to tell you what to do?**

When you're "one down"

Let's take another look at that interaction. This time, we'll make the subordinate active. He's just gotten a request from his supervisor, "I'd like you to head up this project." He's concerned that it'll be busy work. He remembers that every request arises from a need. So, rather than simply saying yes or no, he decides to ask about the need.

Subordinate: Are you saying you're busy and you're looking for some relief from the pile of work you have?

Supervisor: Well, I guess you could put it that way. And I think you could be doing more.

He thinks about his needs and realizes he'd like more interaction with his supervisor on more of a peer level. So, he makes a request that fits more with his own needs.

Subordinate: I'd like to be more involved; I'd just like to choose a project where I could learn more. How about if I take more of a lead on reducing turn around times?

This is just a straightforward application of the ALIVE process. The subordinate takes his supervisor's request as a call for help (**L**isten for a call for help). Rather than refusing, he gets curious about her needs (**I**ntend to connect). He actively confirms her needs (**V**erify what's alive). And he makes a counter- proposal that better meets his needs (**E**ncourage a request that enriches life).

141

Managing Up

After each exchange, write a statement or question that would help draw out the needs behind the supervisor's requests.

Example #1

Caregiver: I'd like you to assign Ricky Stallings to someone else.

Supervisor: Look, just follow through on the assignments I give you.

Caregiver: _____

Example #2

Caregiver: I can't do the enema for Mr. Haskins.

Supervisor: You've become so difficult to schedule. I need you to do what's on your sheet.

Caregiver: _____

Here are some answers we liked:

Example #1

Caregiver: I'd like you to assign Ricky Stallings to someone else.

Supervisor: Look, just follow through on the assignments I give you.

Caregiver: Are you tired of changes around here and need more consistency?

Example #2

Caregiver: I can't do the enema for Mr. Haskins.

Supervisor: You've become so difficult to schedule. I need you to do what's on your sheet.

Caregiver: Are you frustrated with the short staff and need some support to get all the work done?

What do you see?

List three instances you see on the job in which caregivers face challenges with requests. They could include

∴ requests that typically attract "no" in response,

∴ requests that patients or other caregivers hear as demands, or

∴ requests that supervisors make that caregivers would like to renegotiate.

Following each instance, recommend a strategy (using a clarifying request, exploring needs) that could help and suggest a statement or question that can help resolve the challenge.

1. Example of a challenge facing caregivers in your organization

   _____

   _____

   _____

Strategy you'd recommend

❑ use a clarifying request	❑ explore the speaker's needs

How you'd put that strategy into words

_____

_____

_____

2. Example of a challenge facing caregivers in your organization

_____

_____

_____

Strategy you'd recommend

❑ use a clarifying request	❑ explore the speaker's needs

How you'd put that strategy into words

_____

_____

_____

3. Example of a challenge facing caregivers in your organization

_____

_____

_____

Strategy you'd recommend

❑ use a clarifying request	❑ explore the speaker's needs

How you'd put that strategy into words

_____

_____

_____

Bringing it ALIVE

OK, you've seen the steps for taking a compassionate stand. We've been creating reminders to focus your attention on needs: yours, your patients' and your co-workers'. So, you're more likely to get what you want. Very often, all you'll need is a phrase here or there.

Sometimes, you'll notice more resistance than you expect. In those cases, ALIVE can help you negotiate that 'dance,' the give and take of negotiating an interaction. Here's an example.

3 days ago, a 20-month old girl was admitted to a medical floor with fever, cough, and labored breathing. Her viral FA came back showing adenovirus. Yesterday, the senior resident on the case told the intern that he expected the girl to be discharged this morning. When the intern went in to visit the girl this morning, she found the girl wheezing with a temperature of 104 degrees, and the father upset.

Here's a typical interaction between the intern and senior resident before the staff learned the skills.

Senior: I was just by 514.

Intern: I wanted to talk to you about that.

Senior: I also got a call to clear all unneeded beds and hers is one of them.

Intern: I don't think that's a good idea. I really think we should keep her another day.

Senior: Did you miss med school the day they covered viruses?

Intern: No, but you haven't spent the time with her or her father that I have.

Senior: Look, this is exactly what I've been talking to you about, this attitude of yours. Now, I expect you to go do what I asked you to.

It'll come as no surprise that the intern was outraged. In her eyes, the senior resident was on an ego trip at the patient's expense. She wanted to go over his head, and quickly.

If the patient really is in jeopardy, you'll want to follow whatever procedures your Risk Management team has given you. But notice that the patient is still in her bed. The intern may not have to resort to force get her patient the level of care she thinks the girl needs.

It's clear from the start that there isn't high quality rapport between the intern and senior resident. That's a good sign that they could benefit from some active empathy. The ALIVE process could help the intern make some progress without having to escalate.

Assess your rapport

Listen for a call for help

Intend to connect

Verify what's alive

Encourage a request that enriches life

Here's an example of how we coached a physician to use the skills with the senior resident. You'll notice that she adopts the model to her own voice. Also, notice that we don't move straight through the model. We're constantly revisiting steps to refocus our attention and see if we're creating the experience we want.

Senior: Look, this is exactly what I've been talking to you about, this attitude of yours. Now, I expect you to go do what I asked you to.

Coach: (to the intern) Let's pause briefly. I don't get a sense he's hearing you. You don't seem to have the rapport you'd like. Would you agree?

Intern: No, I don't believe his reaction. It's like he's on some ego trip.

Coach: Ok, you've focused so far on the girl. That makes sense; she's your patient. But he's pushing back on that. Maybe he needs something personally. Why don't you try focusing on him a moment?

Intern: You seem pretty ticked off to me.

Senior: You always pull this stuff. Like you don't know you're an intern.

Coach: (to the intern) So, your instinct about him was good. He is mad. There is something he wants.

Intern: Yeah, I can't believe he's making this about me. We've got a patient to deal with.

Coach: (to the intern) That sounds really frustrating. I can see how you'd be concerned for your patient. You want her to get good care. And you want to be taken seriously in your own right.

Intern: Yeah. I do, and he's making it personal.

Coach: (to the intern) Well, you could escalate. Or, since your patient is still in her bed, and you have the guy you need to talk to standing in front of you, can you find a place of curiosity? You might be able to take care of this, right now. What do you think he needs?

Intern: (to the senior) It sounds as though you want some respect, some credit for having been here a few years.

Senior: Yeah, I have been. And let's cut to the chase, I'm your senior.

Coach: (to the intern) So your intuition is right on.

Intern: But that just sets me off. He's messing with my patient because he doesn't like my tone of voice?

Coach: You don't like the behavior you're seeing. Can you focus on the humanity behind it? The need you saw for respect and acknowledgment? Who doesn't want that? Can you let him know how you're feeling and what you want for this girl, remembering that your feelings come out of your own needs?

Intern: (to the senior) You'd like some recognition of the time you've put in and the judgment you've developed. And that translates for you into my discharging this girl.

Senior: That's what I asked you to do.

Intern: I'm having a hard time with this. To be frank, I'm really frustrated. I want to get along with you. I don't want you to think I'm bucking you. At the same time, I'm afraid for this girl. The father said some things to me that scare me for the girl if she goes home. Can you tell me how I can stick up for her in a way that doesn't sound like I'm sticking it to you?

Senior: Yeah, I see what you mean. You gotta have your opinions.

Intern: Would you be willing to come to her room and talk to her Dad?

Senior: I'm not telling you I'm gonna change my mind.

What has the intern accomplished?

The conversation isn't over. We don't know what care the patient needs or what she will receive. The girl is getting a second look. She may benefit from the meeting of two minds, rather than having to settle for the decision one of the physicians could force over the objections of the other.

We see an important shift in the dynamics of the situation. We first thought the patient was in enough jeopardy that we should escalate. In retrospect, we can see that some of that sense of danger came from the intern's own feeling of powerlessness.

The intern has made progress, as well. She stood up for her convictions. She advanced her view of the care she wants for her patient. She did it with a staff member she saw as more powerful and not on her side. And she did it in a way that didn't damage her relationship and might have actually improved it.

Look back over the interaction. As you read it this time, underline the passages that illustrate how the Intern used the ALIVE model to uncover the Senior Resident's needs. In the margin, make notes about how she made progress until she was able to encourage him to revisit the patient's room.

Then, turn the page to see what we thought.

Here's what we saw.

Assess your rapport	**Intern:** No, I don't believe this reaction. It's like he's on some ego trip. The Intern has some strong judgments of the Senior Resident. She sees that they don't share the same concerns and recognizes this as a lack of rapport.
Listen for a call for help	**Coach:** Ok, you've focused so far on the girl. That makes sense; she's your patient. But he's pushing back on that. Maybe he needs something personally. When the coach redirected the Intern's attention to the Senior Resident rather than the patient, he was reminding her to listen for a call for help for the person she was talking to.
Intend to connect	**Coach:** Why don't you try focusing on him a moment? Focusing on the Senior is the first step in connecting.
Verify what's alive in him	**Intern:** You seem pretty ticked off to me. She suggests how the Senior might be feeling.
Intend to Connect	**Coach:** (to the intern) Can you find a place of curiosity? Being curious about someone is the key step in forming an intention to connect with him.

More of what we saw.

Listen for a call for help	**Coach:** What do you think he needs? By looking for the Senior's needs in the midst of his demands, the Intern is looking for how the Senior is asking her to help him.
Verify what's alive in him	**Intern:** (to the senior) It sounds as though you want some respect, some credit for having been here a few years. The Intern is translating her judgments (he's on an ego trip) into the language of needs (he wants some respect and credit).
	Intern: (to the senior) You'd like some recognition of the time you've put in and the judgment you've developed. And that translates for you into my discharging this girl. She adds an effective step, connecting the Senior's request (discharge the girl) to his own needs (some acknowledgement).
Verify what's alive in her	**Intern:** I'm having a hard time with this. To be frank, I'm really frustrated. I want to get along with you. I don't want you to think I'm bucking you. At the same time, I'm afraid for this girl. The father said some things to me that scare me for the girl if she goes home. She's very accountable when she expresses her feelings, needs, and observations. I'm frustrated. I want to get along with you. I don't want you to think this. I'm afraid based on what I heard the father say. So in this step and the previous one, she's framing the entire conversation. She's making it clear in her language that the Senior's requests are connected to his needs and her feelings are connected to her needs and observations.

More of what we saw

Verify what's alive in her	The language above is much clearer and much more likely to arouse compassion than are statements like, "you're on an ego trip, you're making this all about me, and I'm going to escalate!"
Encourage a request that enriches life	**Intern:** Can you tell me how I can stick up for her in a way that doesn't sound like I'm sticking it to you? Now, she makes a very effective request. She recognizes that their argument is much more about the way they have communicated rather than a disagreement in diagnoses. So she makes a request that addresses the immediate problem. She asks for clarification. Notice that he doesn't respond by telling her how she can communicate differently. Instead, he acknowledges the dilemma she's in. But that's progress.
Encourage a request that enriches life	**Intern:** Would you be willing to come to her room and talk to her Dad? He agrees to a request that he may not have agreed to when they met.

Make It Last

The Three Levers of Lasting Change

You've seen how you can use the ALIVE process to take a compassionate stand.

Remember that your needs and beliefs will guide your actions. Your actions will produce results. And you'll compare your results with your needs to decide how you want to invest in creating powerful experiences with patients over time.

Think back over what you've read and the work you've done. You've learned to check in with yourself to gauge your rapport. Listen to your own judgments for a call for help. Set an intention to connect with patients or co-workers. Verify what you feel and need. And encourage a request that will better meet your needs.

You've learned that the inherent power of your position may actually work against you by intimidating others so that you believe you have greater commitment from them than you do. Also, you know that you can work with people you perceive as more or less powerful than you by focusing on needs and making clear your intention that you both get your needs met.

"When the results of my behavior do not meet my needs over time, the problem is a belief."

Linda Eaton
The Galileo
Initiative

Beliefs

What beliefs do you notice still stand in the way of creating powerful interactions with patients or co-workers (Breaker Beliefs)? What beliefs have you developed that will aid you (Booster Beliefs)? And how can you reframe your Breaker Beliefs in other ways that support you?

My Breaker Beliefs

1. _____

2. _____

3. _____

4. _____

5. _____

_____

_____

My Booster Beliefs

1. _____

2. _____

3. _____

4. _____

5. _____

_____

_____

Other ways I can think of my Breaker Beliefs so that they support me.

1. _____

2. _____

3. _____

4. _____

5. _____

_____

Personal practices

We've recommended a set of practices that will help you focus your attention where you're more likely to get what you want. What are some things you can do that will support you in putting the skills to use? Here are some examples we like:

Get a "learning partner," someone you can talk to about what you're doing and can practice the skills with you

Practice makes permanent: repetition of a thought or behavior builds dominant pathways in your brain.

Make commitments to yourself or others about how you'll learn or practice these skills

Put up reminders to yourself about your goals for the day or week or month

Supply yourself with reading and listening material that reinforce the skills and attitudes you want to adopt

What will you do (be as specific as possible):

1. _____

2. _____

3. _____

4. _____

5. _____

Organizational Environment

Look around your organization. What do you notice that helps you create powerful interactions or undermines you?

What would you like to encourage your organization to do? Here are some places to look:

Building policies or strategies that support patients or revising policies that show disregard for them.

1. _____

2. _____

3. _____

Creating signage that reminds you to show support for patients or revising décor that doesn't.

1. _____

2. _____

3. _____

Increasing the topics you handle in internal meetings that foster powerful relationships with patients (for example, sharing stories of great encounters with patients or great encounters the staff has had as customers of any business) or decreasing the time you spend on topics that don't contribute to powerful relationships with patients.

1. _____

2. _____

3. _____

Your Personal Plan

What's next for you?

In each of these three Sections, you've had a chance to record your ideas for creating an environment in which empathy is more visible. Here's your chance to decide the steps you'd like to take. Look over the final unit in your three Sections and collect the ideas that seem most compelling to you. My recommendation is that you don't scrimp. There are two reasons.

The more support you provide yourself, the more quickly, surely, and lastingly you'll affect your life. And what better to fill your life with than reminders of compassion?

Beliefs

The beliefs that I've developed that support me in making empathy visible in my life:

1. _____

2. _____

3. _____

4. _____

5. _____

6. _____

7. _____

8. _____

9. _____

Personal Practices

What I can do personally, to bring empathy more visibly into my life:

What I'll do	When I'll get it done
1. _____ _____	_____/_____/_____
2. _____ _____	_____/_____/_____
3. _____ _____	_____/_____/_____
4. _____ _____	_____/_____/_____
5. _____ _____	_____/_____/_____
6. _____ _____	_____/_____/_____
7. _____ _____	_____/_____/_____

Organizational Environment

How I can influence my environment to bring empathy
more visibly into my organization:

What I'll do	When I'll get it done
1. _____	____/____/____
2. _____	____/____/____
3. _____	____/____/____
4. _____	____/____/____
5. _____	____/____/____
6. _____	____/____/____
7. _____	____/____/____

What does it all add up to?

Some time ago, I was training a diverse group of caregivers. We were working with a scenario that featured an outraged mother. She'd caught three buses to make an appointment and had shown up twenty-five minutes late. We were asking her to reschedule.

She was stomping around swearing at everyone—her daughter, onlookers, and us. "You don't know me!" she shouted, "You may work in this part of town, but you don't know anything about me!" The group was afraid to talk to her.

"This is really terrible for you, isn't it," a nurse finally said, "You really need to know somebody is on your side."

It was as though the mother had been gut-punched. The comment nearly knocked the wind out her. She sat down with tears in her eyes. And we worked out what to do next.

In the debrief that followed, another nurse said, "That's it, that's what patients want most, to know that someone is on their side. That's the most important thing I've heard in this whole training."

And I'd agree with her. That's the long and short.

Of course, you are on your patients' side. We've simply been developing some insights and distinctions, and a vocabulary that will help you make your compassion visible to patients who may have difficulty seeing it, because they're suffering.

It's a framework for doing what you already do when you're at your best.

Some people—like the nurse in the story above—have said that ALIVE gives them a valuable phrase here or there when things get tough. Others have said it's a different way to

interact with people altogether, a way of engaging others instead of dominating them.

Linking empathy skills to patient safety and quality improvement

You'll notice in the scenarios we've covered that the caregivers not only form closer connections to patients. They also uncover information that may impact both their patients' care and the organization's liability.

Consider, for example, the scenario that opened this workbook, the 28 year old Eastern European immigrant and mother of three whose son was diagnosed with Leukemia (p. 17). A nurse we trained discovered that the mother not only felt immensely guilty, she also believed that her son wasn't getting the best possible care because she couldn't afford it and didn't have the English to ask for it.

You may have noted that the woman in the laryngectomy scenario (p. 42) agreed to surgery apparently on little other than her surgeon's say so. And the patient who received an accidental needle stick (p. 51) may have had difficulty distinguishing between a therapist and a nurse.

The incidents in each of these cases don't end with the scenarios. The information that emerged brings up questions about informed consent, and post-surgery decision-making ability.

In these cases, empathy skills create opportunities for caregivers to provide not only a better experience but also better care by creating an environment in which patients feel comfortable revealing relevant personal and medical information.

Multiply the impact of empathy skills by linking them to your patient satisfaction program

Recall the scenario featuring the father of a teen-aged boy recovering after critical care (p. 85). The staff in that unit realized they were currently working with two other families having similar reactions under similar circumstances. In fact, they dealt regularly with families like this who were on edge and responded by micro-managing the care.

By investing in understanding one family well, they developed an approach they could generalize to provide great experiences for other families.

An approach like that can pay off in less stress for staff members and more loyal patients throughout a unit or organization.

Developing a culture of empathy

You might sense that there's a logical next step for these skills and this perspective. It's embodied in the exercises for lasting change at the end of each section.

If ALIVE is a system of "active empathy", a next step is to consider what it would mean to implement a culture of visible empathy or empathy-mindedness.

You'd nurture a culture of visible empathy by making it a practice to ask each other questions such as these:

∴ What needs do our patients have that regularly go unmet?

∴ Which of our policies do we know lead regularly to conflict with patients?

∴ How can we translate what we learn from an interaction with one patient—or a small group of patients—to all the patients we treat?

∴ What needs do our staff members have that regularly go unmet? How can we give ourselves a better experience?

∴ How can we create an abundance of what we need before any of us—patients or staff—suffers?

By nurturing a culture that makes your natural compassion *visible,* you create better experiences for patients and for staff members. And you enhance your organization's reputation for enriching life.

I'm grateful to you for the grace you bring to those who are suffering and for your dedication to enhancing your level of care.

Bibliography

Alpertgood J. Broken appointments. Pediatrics 1964; 34:127-32.

Becker M et al. Predicting mother's compliance with pediatric medical regimens. Med Care 1972; 81:843-54.

Beckman HB, Markakis KM, Suchman AL, Frankel RM. The doctor-patient relationship and malpractice: lessons from plaintiff depositions. Arch Intern Med. 1994;154:1365-1370

Bonder, B., Martin, L., Miracle, A. 2001. Achieving cultural competence: The challenge for clients and healthcare workers in a multicultural society. Generations, 25, 35-42.

Eisenthal S et al. Adherence and the negotiated approach to patienthood. Arch Gen Psychol 1979; 36:393-8.

Hulka B et al. Communication, compliance and concordance between physicians and patients with prescribed medications. Am J Public Health 1976; 66:847-53.

Largest Study of Patient Satisfaction Ever Conducted, by Robert J. Wolosin, Ph.D., Press Ganey Associates, August 2003.

McClure, F. H., and Teyber, E. 1996. "The Multicultural-Relational Approach? In E H. McClure, and E. Teyber, eds., Child and Adolescent Therapy: A Multicultural-Relational Approach.

Medical malpractice as an epidemiological problem, Social Science & Medicine, Volume 59, Issue 1, July 2004, Pages 39-46, Michelle M. Mello and David Hemenway

O'Neil EH. Health Professions Education for the Future: Schools in Service to the Nation. San Francisco, Calif Pew Health Professions Commission; 1993.

Reducing legal risk by practicing patient-centered medicine, Heidi P Forster, Jack Schwartz, Evan DeRenzo. Archives of Internal Medicine. Chicago: Jun 10, 2002. Vol. 162, Iss. 11; pg. 1217, 3 pgs

Rubin, H. J., and Rubin, I. S. 1995. Qualitative Interviewing: The Art of Hearing Data. Thousand Oaks, Calif.: Sage.

Suchman AL, Matthews DA. What makes the patient-doctor relationship therapeutic? exploring the connexional dimension of medical care. Ann Intern Med. 1988;108:125-130

Uhlmann R et al. Relationship of patient request fulfillment to compliance, glycemic control, and other health care outcomes in insulindependent diabetes. J Gen Intern Med 1988; 3:458-63.

Wall Street Journal Online (The), Health Care Poll, Vol. 3, Iss. 19, October 1, 2004

Why is there a Compelling Need for Cultural Competence? The National Center for Cultural Competence. Available at http://gucchd.georgetown.edu/nccc/cultural5.html

A Summary of the ALIVE Process

Listening with Empathy	Taking a Compassionate Stand
Assess your rapport	
Remember that a feeling of unease—whether it originates with your or your patient—is a signal, not to lay back or tip-toe, but to engage in an exchange of empathy.	
Listen for a call for help	
Take your patients' statements as a sign of suffering. Ask yourself, "How can I hear their statements as a call for help?"	Don't resist your judgments. Recognize them as a sign of suffering and ask, **"How can I hear my judgments as a call for help?"**
Intend to connect	
Bracket your agenda, and **get curious** about the experience your patient is having as an end in itself.	Remind yourself that you can get what you need without anyone else being wrong or weaker than you are.
Verify what's alive	
Focus your attention on your patient's feelings and needs, right now.	Focus your attention on what you feel and need in this moment.
Encourage a request that enriches life	
Suggest a concrete action you and your patient might use to meet your patient's needs.	Suggest a concrete action that would help meet your needs.

About Tim Dawes

Tim Dawes is President and Founder of Interplay, Inc., as well as a consultant, trainer, and executive coach. His unique perspective comes from conducting custom trainings for hospitals, healthcare and social work trade associations, and university courses. The step-by-step process Interplay teaches helps care givers to increase revenue and decrease liability for their organizations by creating excellent experiences for patients and themselves. Interplay's training is based on Compassionate Communication (some call it nonviolent communication or NVC), originally developed by Marshall Rosenberg, PhD. NVC is a process for creating compassionate connection—not just communications—that's been field-tested internationally for over 45 years. The training technology Interplay uses—live standardized scenarios—was developed over the course of six years and in more than 500 education and training sessions at a major university.

To inquire into retaining Interplay for live training, find special reports, mini-courses, materials for purchase, or to sign-up for monthly "how to" articles, see Mr. Dawes's website www.interplaygroup.com.